LOW-IMPACT SWIMMING POOL EXERCISES

For People with Injuries, Limited Movement, and Seniors

Evelyn Turner, Author

Jenifer Caccia, Illustrator

Table of Contents

Introduction

I t is all too easy to make excuses that encourage you to skip out on exercise. You might say to yourself, "I'm too old to work out like I used to and it's too difficult, so why bother?" or "my injury or chronic pain means that workouts that involve running and weightlifting just aren't possible for me." While it is true that old age, injury, and limited mobility can all make traditional workouts more difficult, this does not mean you have to stop exercising entirely, nor does it negate the need for regular exercise to keep you fit and healthy.

The many benefits of exercise, including its ability to promote heart health, improve your mood, and assist with weight loss, are important for people of all ages and physical conditions. In fact, if you are older or if you have an injury or disability that makes it harder to be active on a daily basis, committing to a light workout becomes even more important. But high-impact exercises like running, jumping jacks, and playing sports can be prohibitively difficult in your condition. You may not be able to complete these exercises without pain, and if your workout routine is hurting you, it is doing more harm than good. Excessive joint pain can indicate that your workout is doing damage to your muscles and bones, which can be a serious problem if old age or injury limits your recovery.

Of course, this does not mean you cannot exercise. You just need to focus on low-impact workouts that are easier on your joints. This is where swimming pool exercises come in. Working out in a swimming pool relieves pressure on your joints and keeps you from making sharp, jarring movements that could otherwise lead to further injury. You can stay active without the risk of hurting yourself, which will in turn help you look and feel your best. Regularly exercising in the pool can gradually increase the strength of your muscles over time while also improving your cardiovascular health.

If you are unfamiliar with exercising in a pool, do not worry. You do not have to be an Olympic swimmer to follow along with the exercises included in this book, though you should be comfortable in water to perform these exercises safely. In *Low-Impact Swimming Pool Exercises*, you will learn not just how to work out in the pool, but also the components of exercise that will ensure your workouts are as effective as possible without putting excess tension on any area of your body. Practicing regular pool exercises will make you more flexible, improve your balance, strengthen your muscles, and expand your range of motion.

I know just how useful swimming pool exercises can be from personal experience. I have always been passionate about exercise, but after I was injured while in the service, it became incredibly difficult to practice the same exercises as I did before. Using an elliptical machine was the closest I could come to exercising without pain, though even this still became painful if I tried to make it a regular habit. I was at a loss until I turned my attention to low-impact exercises, and swimming pool exercises in particular. Pool exercises do not exacerbate my injuries. They let me experience all the benefits of exercise without any of the pain or muscle damage, which encouraged me to return to a daily workout routine. I want to help you achieve these same benefits by opening your eyes to a new pain-free way to stay fit.

Do not let worries or excuses hold you back from embracing the perfect exercise plan for you. It is true that you should avoid jumping blindly into a new, demanding workout program when you have an injury, so you do not make that injury worse. But when you work out in the pool following the guided exercises within this book, you can avoid potentially harmful exercises and instead stick to only the ones best suited for your current circumstances. If you ever feel pain during an exercise, stop, reassess your form, and make necessary adjustments. Any exercises you attempt from this book should be completely pain-free. Do only what you can in the beginning. This may not seem like a lot at first if you have not worked out in a while, but over time your strength and stamina will increase. Before long, you will be doing more than you ever thought possible.

Pool exercises are the perfect middle ground between grueling workouts that leave you sweaty and exhausted, and lazing on the couch without exercising at all. Make exercise fun and stress-free again by jumping in the pool today and experience the benefits of swimming pool exercises for yourself.

CHAPTER 1

Why Exercise?

I f you are not someone who typically finds the time to fit a workout into your daily schedule, you might feel a little hesitant to start any type of exercise, let alone something that could turn into a program. After all, you are not going to become a professional athlete, and you are likely not exactly in your glory days either. Is it really necessary for you to exercise if you are not concerned about your athletic ability?

The truth is that the more issues you have with mobility, the more important it is for you to make exercise a routine part of your schedule. As you age, or as an injury or health condition starts to affect your muscles and joints, you start to lose your usual range of motion. Performing regular tasks can cause pain because you are not used to stretching these muscles. You are also in more danger of injuring yourself, even from small missteps and impacts. Something as simple as missing a stair could result in a sprained ankle or worse, and this likelihood only increases the less you work your muscles and joints.

Even though exercising may be harder, it is more important than ever before that you are seriously committed to staying active in whatever way you can. Of course, this does not mean you have to be ready to run a mile at a moment's notice. It just means that you should commit to some low-impact workout routines, like those that can be accomplished in the pool, at least once every few days to keep your body in top condition.

Remember that all the work you are putting in is for the sake of your health. If you want to remain in good physical shape and make sure you can continue taking care of yourself no matter your age or range of movement, you need to exercise frequently. Jumping in the pool is the perfect way to address your body's needs without putting too much strain on yourself.

Improving Your Physical Fitness

The more you work out, the stronger you become. This is true for super-athletes just as much as it is true for the regular Joe. Routine exercise is a very important step in keeping yourself physically fit in many different areas. These include your mobility, balance, strength, posture, and general fitness, all of which will help you navigate your everyday life and support a healthy, happy lifestyle.

Mobility

Your mobility is your capacity for unrestricted movement, especially in regard to your flexibility. This is primarily an issue with your joints, which can start to lock up and restrict your ability to get around. Mobility issues are easy to spot, as you will notice them interfering with your ability to perform regular activities like stretching to grab something off the top shelf in the kitchen or bending down to tie your shoes. You may also experience joint pain when sitting or lying down, as well as when you are standing up.

Some mobility issues are caused by injuries that do not heal property, but many people also experience these issues as they age. This is because of changes in your ligaments, which connect bones at your joints. As you get older, your ligaments become less flexible, shortening slightly if you do not use them frequently. Additionally, aging can impact the cartilage and lubricating fluid, known as synovial fluid, that helps cushion your joints. As you continue to age, "joint movement becomes stiffer and less flexible because the amount of lubricating fluid inside your joints decreases and the cartilage becomes thinner" (Better Health Channel, 2015, para. 9). Without the added cushion, bending at the joints becomes more difficult.

Certain health conditions commonly associated with aging can also negatively impact your mobility. For example, rheumatoid arthritis causes inflammation and swelling in your joints, which makes it harder to bend them. Osteoarthritis speeds up the process of cartilage breakdown, resulting in stiffness. Osteoporosis makes it more likely for you to experience an injury because your bones lose their density, gradually becoming more brittle.

These conditions can all limit your range of motion, but you can undo their effects with some low-impact exercises. By working your joints, you promote better synovial fluid flow and reduce the rate at which your cartilage deteriorates.

Exercise also helps strengthen your bones and builds muscle mass, which makes it easier for you to contract and relax your muscles. If you make a point to keep moving, you can avoid stiff joints and other issues that contribute to reduced mobility.

Balance

Balance comes from your lower body, including your legs, lower back, and stomach muscles, also known as your core. Trouble with balancing can be especially dangerous as you get older, as a fall is more likely to result in injury. Therefore, it is important to perform low-impact exercises that strengthen the muscles in your lower body and help you maintain your balance as you go about your day.

Just about every activity that involves movement in some way will help you train the muscles involved in improving your balance. Even something as easy as going for a walk on a regular basis can make a big difference, though more complex exercises like yoga are often associated with balance training. Luckily, if your limited mobility prevents you from doing yoga, you can still receive these benefits from pool exercises. In the pool, the water assists in keeping you upright and alleviates tension in your muscles, while the gentle movement of the water ensures you are engaging your leg and core muscles to stay standing or treading water. With repeated exercise, you can greatly improve your balance and reduce the risk of harmful falls.

Strength

Physical strength is important for much more than just lifting heavy objects. For one, when you build your strength in your muscles, you are less likely to get tired from performing everyday activities. You will also minimize the risk of being seriously injured from regular bumps and bruises, as stronger muscles provide greater cushion around your bones. Improving your physical strength can help you feel more confident and proud of how you look as well, which can benefit your mental health as well by raising your self-esteem.

Despite all of its benefits, many people avoid exercises that focus on strength training because these workouts are very difficult if you have limited mobility. You likely cannot lift a heavy weight if you are out of practice and are experiencing other issues due to age or injury, and even a simple push-up can become incredibly tough if you cannot yet support your body weight. Still, there are plenty of ways you can build muscle mass over time even if you do not have very much right now, and these methods include pool exercises. When you perform strength training workouts in the pool, you will find that it is easier to lift weights and perform repetitive motions because the water takes some of the stress off your joints. You will also be engaging your whole body when you are in the water, not just your arm or back muscles, as is the case with most standard weightlifting. This means you are getting a more full-body workout, and you can build strength in many areas at the same time.

Posture

Bad posture can have much more serious repercussions than a tendency to slouch. When you continually practice poor posture, you put a significant amount of strain on your muscles. This frequently leads to stiffness and soreness and further limits your mobility, but it can have other, more long-lasting negative effects as well. For example, frequently leaning and putting large amounts of weight on one of your joints can deteriorate your ability to flex that joint normally. You may experience nerve pain or damage that results in a tingly, numb feeling and an inability to move your limbs properly. In some cases, posture issues can create spinal dysfunctions, and you may become unable to fully bend over or straighten your back.

It is important to make a conscious effort to practice good posture whenever possible, and exercise can assist with this goal. Your core muscles have the greatest influence on your posture, as they are engaged in torso movements as well as supporting your spine when you are in an upright, neutral position. The more you strengthen your core, the better your control over your posture will be, and the less effort you will have to put into remembering not to hunch your shoulders or lean to one side.

Overall Physical Fitness

In addition to the more specific benefits that exercise provides in terms of mobility, balance, strength, and posture, regular exercise is a key part of keeping yourself healthy. It helps you burn excess body fat when used alongside proper nutrition. It also supports cardiovascular health. Exercise keeps your heart pumping, ensures your lungs are functioning optimally, and keeps your blood pressure at a safe level. It can be tempting to avoid exercising entirely when it is not as easy to stay active as it used to be, but given its many benefits, there are plenty of reasons to make sure you are getting at least a minor workout in every day.

Luckily, you do not need to spend all your time in the gym to achieve a healthy level of fitness. In fact, you may not need to exercise very much each day as long as you make sure you are performing the right kinds of workouts. The trick is to incorporate "isotonic exercise — activities that use your large muscle groups in a rhythmic, repetitive fashion without making your muscles work against heavy resistance" (Harvard Health Publishing, 2009, para. 8). As you might imagine, pool exercises fit this description perfectly, so they make the ideal addition to your regular routine if you want to create and maintain healthy habits.

Exercising in the Water

There are plenty of reasons to get active, but you might still be wondering what benefits exercising in the pool can provide. Pool workouts can be some of the most effective options for people with limited mobility, so it is frequently recommended by physicians and personal trainers. It provides incredible benefits to common aches and pains that arise when you get older, such as joint stiffness and an inability to rest at night. Additionally, working out in the pool helps you feel less like you are sweating it out at the gym and more like you are just having fun, which can make it much easier to stick to a workout routine.

Limit Your Risk of Falling

When you are young, falling is not such a big deal, but as you get older it can become a cause for concern. For one, your balance may decrease with age and a lack of physical activity, so you are more prone to falling in the first place. For another, your bones become less dense over time, so there is a higher risk of fracturing or even breaking a bone after a fall. You may also struggle to get up on your own, and if you live alone, this can be a scary thought. These issues are only worsened if you have an injury that further limits your ability to get around, or if you have undergone a serious surgical procedure that makes it more difficult for your body to focus on balance before a fall and recovery after one.

Pool exercises can minimize this risk by improving your balance, which helps you catch yourself before a fall and limits the possibility of injury. These exercises also improve your posture, which means you will find yourself overbalancing less often. Additionally, they support muscle strength, so if you do fall, you are less likely to experience a serious injury as a result. Exercising frequently in the pool ensures you can navigate the world safely, no matter your age or current condition.

Reduce Impact on Your Joints

High-impact exercises can be especially dangerous for people with joint pain and stiffness. If you are not careful about what kind of workouts you practice, you could end up aggravating your joints rather than relieving issues with them. Many workouts that involve rapid, jerky movements or that jolt your body, such as those that involve exercise machines or even simply going for a run, should be avoided. Too many high-impact workouts can actually increase your risk of stress fractures and other injuries. One study of 45- to 55-year-olds tracked joint pain in high-impact and low-impact workouts and found that "people in the high-activity group had much more damage, including cartilage and ligament lesions and buildup of fluid in the bone marrow, than those in the low-activity group," with "93% of people in the high-activity groups [suffering] cartilage damage vs. 60% in the low-activity group" (Laino, 2009, para. 13). Of course, this does not mean that you should give up on exercise entirely, but it does mean that you should be cautious about how you choose to exercise.

If you have trouble with your joints, working out in the pool can greatly reduce the effects of high-impact exercises. Even if you have arthritis or osteoporosis, you will find that it is much easier for you to move in the water. As previously mentioned, water reduces the tension on your joints as you move, making it easier to lift your arms and kick your feet. This means you can perform a full exercise routine without experiencing severe joint pain afterward, and you may feel less sore overall as well. Making sure to move your joints can also minimize the effects of arthritis and alleviate joint pain, so it is definitely worth the extra effort.

Strengthening Your Muscles

Many people work out with high-intensity exercises and heavy weights in an effort to bulk up. You may not be able to complete such strenuous exercises, and you may not have any desire to become a bodybuilder either, but low-impact pool exercises can still help you increase muscle mass to provide extra cushion and protection. The stronger your muscles are, the easier it will be for you to perform regular daily activities, and the less you will have to worry about falling and getting hurt, as mentioned earlier.

Pool workouts primarily target your core, arm, and leg muscles, though muscles from all over your body are also involved in keeping you stable in the water. When you engage these muscle groups, you can reverse the gradual decline of your muscle mass that often occurs with age and inactivity. You will also increase the protection around your bones, leading to fewer fractures. Exercise has the added benefit of increasing bone density as well, reducing the effects of osteoporosis and related conditions. You can support this process by ensuring you are getting adequate amounts of vitamin D and calcium. Changing your diet can improve your intake of both of these nutrients, though you can also raise your vitamin D levels by spending more time outside in the sun.

Improving Sleeping Habits

If you tend to toss and turn at night, unable to shut your eyes and fall asleep, exercise can be the perfect solution to this problem. This is because exercise wears you out, in a good way. When you work out, your body needs to rest to repair your muscles and provide you with adequate energy. For most people, adding a pool workout to their daily routine means they will feel sufficiently tired by the end of the day, and they can drift off right away. Getting adequate amounts of sleep is very important for your body's ability to function regularly, and when you find yourself going to bed earlier, you will also find that you wake up with greater levels of energy to tackle the rest of your day.

While exercise can make you sleepy, it can also help revitalize you if you find your eyelids are slipping shut halfway through the day. This is because a workout gets your blood pumping, which helps to keep you awake and alert. Avoid drinking too much caffeine, which can cause a spike in your blood pressure, and try some light exercise for a quick pick-me-up that does not ruin your ability to fall asleep at night.

Having Fun

Finally, one of the best reasons to choose pool exercises over other kinds of workouts is because they hardly feel like workouts at all. Many people give up on improving their fitness because they aren't naturally inclined to get much pleasure out of working out. They know all the benefits, but trying to jog for more than a few minutes, or spending time at the gym lifting weights, sounds like a nightmare. Workouts can be strenuous and even boring if there is no other stimulus involved, which discourages people from keeping up with their routine. The same is not true of pool exercises, which are more engaging and tend to feel more fun than standard exercise routines.

When you are in the pool, you are more likely to have a positive outlook toward exercise, as you feel like you're simply having a good time splashing around in the water. If you want to really take the 'work' out of 'workout,' invite some friends along and exercise together. The more fun you can make your workouts, the more likely you are to stick with them, and the more you will get to enjoy the associated benefits.

CHAPTER 2

Pool Safety

E xercising in the pool is often safer than exercising on the ground for people with limited mobility, as there is less of a risk of falling or pulling a muscle. Still, it is important to understand the basic practices that ensure you have a safe experience when you get in the water. Learn about how you can keep yourself safe in the pool so you can focus your energy on working out.

In addition to the rules, you should follow when you are in the water, keep in mind common safety measures that apply to any kind of workout. While you do want to push yourself to stay active, and this sometimes means engaging in more strenuous activity, a great workout should never put you in danger. Do not push yourself to continue if you ever feel like you are putting yourself at risk performing a given exercise, or if you feel any sort of pain from a certain pose or repetitive movement. Stop, double check your form, and see if the pain is resolved. If not, stop the exercise and wait until you are well-rested enough to try again without hurting yourself, or until support arrives if the problem is serious. When exercising, you should always put your safety first, which means following pool safety rules and more general good practices for exercise, which we will discuss in greater detail in the next chapter.

Rules of the Pool

Think of basic pool safety like a set of rules laid out by a lifeguard. You want to adhere to these rules because they are your best bet for reducing the risk of accidentally doing something dangerous and hurting yourself. These rules include knowing how to swim, working out with a partner, using the edge of the pool to support yourself, and staying in a water depth that is most comfortable for you.

Know How to Swim

This might seem a little obvious, but if you want to work out in the water, you should be a fairly proficient swimmer. You do not have to be on the Olympic swim team, but you should at least be able to comfortably tread water, hold your breath for a few seconds, and find your way back to the surface when you are underwater. Many people believe that as long as they can stand up in the pool, they do not really need to know how to swim. However, while you may not need to go underwater for most exercises, being unable to swim while in the pool, or lacking confidence in your swimming abilities, can actually put you in a great deal of danger.

There is a risk that while you are exercising, you might overbalance or slip and end up going underwater. If you are not expecting it, the feeling can be disorienting, especially if you are already tired from your workout or if you happened to injure yourself. You may panic at first, leaving you unable to find your footing. If you are a confident swimmer, these feelings of panic will quickly fade, and you will be able to right yourself and return to the surface quickly. If not, you may be unable to react appropriately, which could make it hard to think clearly and get yourself to safety. Therefore, you should be comfortable with swimming before you decide to start working out in the pool. If you do not yet have your swimming skills down, take some time to practice, then return to this book when you are ready.

Partner Up

If you have the option, it is best to swim around other people rather than going in the pool by yourself. Ideally, you might go to the pool to swim and exercise with a group of friends, but even having other swimmers at a community pool is better than swimming alone. This is because if you are ever disoriented or injured to the point that you need assistance, someone else can call for help and get you out of the pool. The problem could be as minor as a muscle cramp or as major as an unfortunately timed heart attack, but whatever it is, you'll want someone else around if anything happens.

The good news is that partnering up comes with the added benefit of making exercise a little more engaging. When you work out with friends, you are more likely to stay motivated and stick to your regimen, and you also have people to hold you accountable for maintaining your workout schedule. Group settings are great for exercise, even if you take a class with a bunch of strangers, because you all end up helping

15

each other and feeding into each other's positive energies just by being nearby. Grab a buddy before you hit the pool, and you will find it easier to stay active overall.

Hold the Edge

When you are first learning how to perform different workouts in the pool, it is a good idea to stick close to the steps or ladder while still giving yourself enough space to fully complete the motions. You can hold onto the edge and perform the exercises a few times, so you get a good feel for the different workouts. You do not have to use the edge forever, but this method has a few benefits when you are just starting out. For one, it allows you to focus on the movement and your posture without worrying about the water displacing you, which makes it easier for you to get the hang of things. For another, keeping a hand on the edge ensures that if you slip, have a cramp, or experience anything else that might normally cause you to lose your footing, you can hold the edge and keep your head above the water. This way, you will be safer, and you will have less trouble maintaining your balance when you are learning and performing your exercises.

After a while, you will get enough practice to have the moves down and develop your "sea legs" well enough to stand on your own. At this point, you can let go of the edge and give yourself a little more space, though it is still a good idea to stay near the ladder just in case.

Avoid Water That Is Too Deep

One common mistaken belief held by people who are new to working out in the pool is that it is best to do all exercises in deeper waters. In truth, there are many workouts that can be performed perfectly well in more shallow waters. There are some exercises where the water level needs to be a little higher, but you do yourself no favors by trying to force yourself to perform these more difficult workouts sooner than you're ready for them. Try them a few times in the shallow end of the pool to get the basic movements down, and do not worry about incorporating them into your regular routine until you feel like you're ready to progress.

Your comfort level at different depths will vary with your swimming skill level and your physical fitness. If you are still a little uncertain in the water, it is best to remain at the shallow end so there is little to no risk of danger to you. As you gradually become a better swimmer, and as you become more well-versed in the different exercises, you will start to have fewer reservations about swimming and working out in the deep end. At this point, you can begin to move further toward the deeper parts of the pool, as you will have the confidence and prowess necessary to keep yourself safe without issues.

Overall, the most important rule when working out in the pool is to prioritize your safety. It is okay to push yourself, but this should never come at the expense of your long-term wellbeing. If you find that a certain workout is outside of your comfort zone, put a pin in it and come back to it later when you have strengthened your muscles, improved your balance, and gotten a little more comfortable in the water. This is not just a good way to approach pool exercises; it is a good way to approach exercises of any kind.

CHAPTER 3

Personal Safety

Maintaining your pool safety is very important, but it is just one part of the proper protocols for a safe and productive exercising environment. The other key aspect is ensuring your personal safety. Workouts can be strenuous and working out improperly can undo all the benefits that routine exercises normally provide. In fact, points of concern like using bad form and overworking yourself can actually increase your risk of injury, in some cases further limiting your mobility. You want to focus on making forward progress when you work out, and this means putting your safety first so you can ensure you do not waste all the effort you are putting into improving your physical health.

Be Aware of Your Limits

Everyone has physical limitations, and if you are older or have a condition that prevents you from moving regularly, your limits are going to be even more restrictive than those of an average person. Yes, exercise should help you improve your physical capabilities to an extent, but it is counterproductive to attempt to accomplish this by ignoring the existence of your limits. If you do not take care to pace yourself and make progress according to your own speed, you might hurt yourself, or at the very least discourage yourself from continuing with your new workout program.

Rid yourself of the idea that your current physical limits are something to be ashamed of. It is good to make improvements to your mobility, balance, strength, and other skills, but there is nothing wrong with not being quite as fit as you were decades ago. Aging is a natural process, and mobility limitations caused by chronic conditions or injuries cannot be miraculously overcome with willpower. It is only by understanding your limitations that you can create a proper fitness routine that accounts for them without causing you any pain.

You might have heard the phrase "no pain, no gain" before in reference to exercise, but taking this phrase too literally can spell trouble. Exercise should never cause you pain. If your muscles hurt when you are working out, you are likely pushing yourself too hard. This is a good indicator that it is time for a break. The worst thing you can do if you feel pain is to keep exercising at the same intensity as before, as this will only make the pain worse and increase your risk of really injuring yourself. Instead, try to lower the intensity of your workout, and check in with yourself frequently so you know whether it is safe to continue exercising or if you need to take a break.

Warning Signs for Low-Impact Workouts

Many workouts are created with the goal of getting your heart pumping and your pulse racing, but these are generally workouts intended for people with very few physical limitations. Pool exercises are meant to be performed at a slower pace and cause less strain on your body. You should not feel like your heart is about to beat out of your chest after performing too many reps. If your heart is racing, this is a strong sign that you need to ease up a little and give yourself space to breathe, or you could end up pushing yourself too hard.

Low-impact exercises also should not make you sweat profusely, nor should they interfere with your ability to breathe regularly. If you are breathing heavily or if you feel a tightness in your chest when you try to perform the exercises, this is a sign that you should try something a little easier and work your way up to more difficult exercises. You do not have to go for the most exhausting workouts right away, and if any exercise does not seem like it is safe for you, it is best to take a break and choose a different one for the time being.

Finally, pay careful attention to any feelings of faintness, dizziness, weakness, or lightheadedness that might arise from your workout routine. If you experience any of these symptoms, leave the pool and let your body rest for a few moments. You may have hit your limit for the day, and that is okay. Everyone builds muscle and stamina at their own pace, and it is important to listen to your body when you are working out. Exhausting yourself is not going to help you improve your overall fitness, and your workouts should not leave you on the verge of passing out or getting sick. Be kind to yourself and give yourself time to gradually expand your limits with repeated exercise.

Take Rests

Knowing and respecting your limits means taking breaks when you need them. You do not want to keep working the same area over and over, even if you want to build muscle specifically in one area. Ideally, you want to have a more even distribution of added muscle, and the best way to achieve this is to avoid overworking any one area. Let yourself rest when you need it and return to working out when you feel like you can handle it again.

Resting does not necessarily mean you have to stop working out entirely. You can rest one area of your body just by moving on to an exercise that targets another area. For example, if you are exercising your right arm, you can allow that arm to rest by shifting to focus on your left arm instead. This way, you keep yourself moving without straining the muscles of one arm. You can also take a quick break in between these two workouts to ensure you can tackle the left arm exercises with the same enthusiasm and energy as you had when you started the right arm ones. If you are performing a workout that engages both arms at the same time, take a brief rest and then move on to something that works your legs or the core of your body instead. Give your body time to heal so you can keep giving it your all.

Hydrate

You might be surrounded by water, but this does not lessen the need for you to stay hydrated while you work out. Your body's cells need water to properly function, especially the cells and tissues that make up your muscles. Proper hydration "regulates your body temperature and lubricates your joints," and it "helps transport nutrients to give you energy and keep you healthy" (American Academy of Family Physicians, 2020, para. 1) so you can avoid exhaustion and muscle cramps. The best way to supply your body with the water it needs is by drinking before, during, and after your workout. Since you are not performing any high-intensity workouts, water should be fine, and you can avoid consuming the added sugars that come with sports drinks.

Hydration is especially important when you are in the pool because you are not sweating to the same extent you would be during other exercises. If you are working out on land, in the sun on a hot day, you can feel yourself get sweaty. This reminds you that your body is losing water, and that you need to keep drinking to replenish it. When you are in the pool, you tend to sweat less, and any sweat you do produce gets wicked away by the water. Therefore, you may not realize how much water you are losing, which means replenishing your body's fluids might slip your mind.

Create Reminders

To make hydration easier for yourself, make sure to always have water on hand. Fill up a large, reusable plastic or metal bottle before you go to the pool and leave it within your line of sight. Just moving the bottle closer to you can subconsciously remind you of the need to stay hydrated, and if you do not have to get out of the pool to get a drink, you are more likely to take a few sips in between exercises.

Typically, working up a sweat will naturally make you a little more thirsty, but if you still have trouble drinking regularly you might find it easier if you flavor your water with some cut-up fruit. A few slices of strawberries or lemons can make plain old tap water much more appealing so you can ensure you are drinking enough during your workout.

Moderate Your Exertion

Many people believe that an exercise must be exhausting to be effective, but this just is not true. Any sort of physical movement is good for you and getting too worn out by a single exercise can actually be a sign you are pushing yourself too hard and sabotaging your progress. You should be able to comfortably perform eight repetitions, or reps, of a given exercise. If you cannot complete all eight without feeling out of breath or being in pain, adjust the exercise so you decrease your exertion level.

There are many ways to lower the exertion you experience from a certain exercise. First, try exercising at a less demanding level, usually by making the workout a little less intense. If you apply less force and take things slower, you can usually turn a strenuous exercise into a more approachable one. Keep your movements steady and controlled and avoid jerking your arms or legs. These more controlled movements ensure you are not exhausting yourself for minimal results. Better yet, slowing things down helps you perfect your form. When you get enough practice and

24

you eventually feel ready to increase your pace slightly, you can do so knowing you are using perfect form, which helps you get the greatest benefit out of the exercise with the lowest risk of injury.

If the exercise in question involves water weights, try doing it without the weight at first. Just move your arms through the exercise on their own. This decreases the amount of resistance you experience from the water, making it much easier on your muscles. When you feel like you have the moves down and you are no longer exerting yourself, you can try it out with the weights. As the exercise becomes easy with a light weight you can increase the intensity of the exercise when you are ready by switching to a medium weight and then eventually a heavy weight.

You can also reduce water resistance by moving out of the deep end of the pool and doing your workouts in a mid-level depth or even a shallow area. If less of your body is submerged, you are not pushing against the water with every movement. For example, if all of your arms (up to the shoulder) are below the water, it is going to require much more force for you to lift up a weight. However, if about half of your arm is out of the water, you can freely move your biceps and triceps while still getting the added benefits of the water for your lower arms, core, and legs. The deeper you are, the more water surrounds your body, and the more intense your workout will be. Moving to more shallow waters allows you to practice an exercise a few times without wearing yourself out.

If all else fails, try cutting down on the number of reps you are performing. If you cannot quite make it to eight reps without tiring yourself out, try six, or whatever number you are comfortable with. For more demanding exercises, you may have to start with just two or three reps at a time and slowly work your way up to a higher rep count. It is okay if you cannot handle doing so many reps right away. With practice, you will become more capable, and the workouts will get easier for you, so you can tackle the ones that previously gave you so much trouble without issue. Once you reach a rep count you are comfortable with, you can add an extra rep or two whenever you feel you are ready until you can complete a full eight count.

Pay Attention to Your Breathing

Your breathing rhythm is the best indicator of how hard you are working and how much strain your body is under. If you are breathing very heavily, or if your breaths are shallow and do not feel like they are filling your lungs, this is a sign you are overworking yourself. Make sure to take measured, deep breaths as you work out. The best method is to breathe with the same rhythm as your workout.

As you start each exercise, take a deep breath in. When you reach the apex of the exercise, your lungs should feel full. Then, as you move to return to the starting position, slowly and steadily release this breath. Each rep should be one full breath, in and out. Carefully counting your breaths like this will ensure you avoid holding your breath during a workout, which could deprive your body of the oxygen it needs. This also makes it easier to maintain control over your movements during your workout. Everything should be carefully measured so your workout is safe and efficient.

CHAPTER 4

Flotation and Resistance Devices

Many exercises can be performed without any equipment at all, but some require special gear. This is especially important for pool exercises, where various flotation and resistance devices can help you get a more beneficial workout. Flotation devices help stabilize you in the water. This allows you to focus your efforts on your form and the reps you are completing, making it easier for you to get used to the exercises when you are just starting out. Resistance devices, on the other hand, are meant to make your workouts a little more challenging. They make it feel like they add some extra weight, and they can be incorporated once you can complete the exercises on your own to make your workout even more effective.

Throughout the book, you will occasionally see these flotation and resistance devices mentioned if they can be used with a certain exercise. As you become more familiar with the exercises and with your abilities, you may also discover additional ways to use these devices. Use them to your

27

advantage so you can get the most out of the time you spend in the pool.

Flotation Belt

A flotation belt is a belt made of EVA foam and another waterproof material, typically nylon. It is similar to wearing a life jacket or arm floats, but with the added benefit of being able to wrap it around your waist and buckle it in place so it does not inhibit your ability to perform any exercises. Flotation belts are generally more comfortable and more suited to the pool environment than many other flotation devices that are primarily designed for an ocean or lake setting, or that are typically made for kids who are just learning to swim.

Flotation belts offer additional support to perform exercises in the deeper end of the pool even if you are not a strong swimmer. They let you put your full focus on learning and performing the exercise itself rather than worrying about keeping yourself afloat. Not only does this better allow you to work out, but it can also help build up your confidence when you are just starting out in the pool. While the belt is used for flotation purposes first and foremost, there are some exercises where having a belt wrapped around your waist can add a little resistance too, which can make the belt a good tool to keep around even when you have improved your swimming capabilities.

Using a flotation belt is not required for any of the exercises covered in this book, and it will not be mentioned explicitly. It is up to you to decide whether or not you need the device and when you should use it. Many people find that it's worth the investment if they are not great swimmers, but you may want to try out a few exercises first and then see if you need the assistance of a flotation device or not.

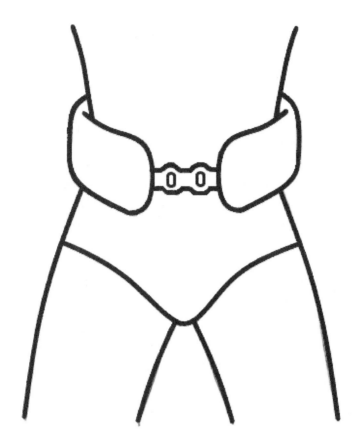

Pool Noodles

Pool noodles are tubes of buoyant foam that can be used as flotation devices in the pool. Pool noodles have three main purposes. These are balance, exercise, and flotation. You may be more familiar with them as pool toys, but they can be incorporated into exercises as well. In addition to assisting with flotation, pool noodles can help you keep yourself balanced in the pool, which provides added security. They may be used for some exercises in the pool, though very few of the workouts discussed in this book address exercising with a noodle. Instead, it is mainly for balance and self-confidence purposes, though workout routines discussed in other books may make more use of them.

For Balance

It is easy to feel a little off-balance in the water, especially if there are other people in the pool with you. If you already have limited mobility, these balance issues are exacerbated until the workouts start improving your balance. In the meantime, you can use a pool noodle for assistance.

When you are in the pool, lay the pool noodle on the surface of the water in front of your chest, horizontal so the ends stick out to either side of you. Then tuck the right side under your right arm, allowing that end of the noodle to stick out behind you. Repeat this on the left side so the noodle curves around your chest with its end protruding behind you as well. As you walk toward the deep end of the pool, the noodle should remain on or near the surface of the water, and it should be comfortably wedged under your arms. This way, the very top of your torso as well as your neck and head will remain above the water, and the pool noodle should stay in place to help maintain your balance. You should have little trouble raising one leg at a time, so it is easier to build up your sense of balance when you use the noodle for support.

For Exercise

Pool noodles can be used to increase resistance. If you position a pool noodle under your arm and then hold a weight in your hand, the pool noodle's support will make it easier to lift the weight toward the surface, but also adds resistance when bringing the weight back down. You can also perform workouts that involve attempting to push the noodle under the water in a steady and controlled manner, then slowly bringing it back up. You can even use pool noodles for added resistance when performing underwater lunges. Use the buoyancy of the noodle to your advantage to improve your workout.

For Flotation

The usage you may be most familiar with for pool noodles is as a flotation device. As mentioned earlier, you can use the noodle to keep your upper body out of the water, which assists in both balance and flotation. Additionally, you can bend the noodle under you and sit on it, which will allow you to remain upright while freeing up your legs.

Whatever purpose you use them for, pool noodles, like flotation belts, can be used in both long-term and short-term contexts. When you are first starting out, exercising with a pool noodle can help you learn the basic movements without the fear that you will lose your balance and go underwater. Later on, you can incorporate them into certain exercises once you feel like you can stay afloat on your own.

Bar Float

A bar float looks similar to a long barbell that weight lifters use when working out. The bar float is around 27 inches long, is thin and hollow with round ends and are made of foam. Rather than weighing you down, they float on the surface, and can therefore be a useful tool for stabilizing yourself during workouts. This allows you to move away from the edge of the pool but still have something to rest your weight on to improve your balance. It functions similarly to grabbing a handle while you are working out to keep yourself in place. In addition to assisting with balance, the bar float can also increase your confidence and help you feel more secure while moving in the pool.

The bar float is not directly referenced in any of the exercises in this book. However, you can choose to use it as a hand hold if you like.

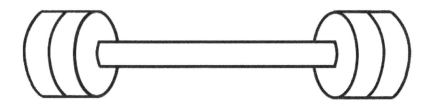

Water Dumbbell

Water dumbbells look similar to the dumbbells a weightlifter uses when working out. However, they have a plastic bar with foam on the ends. They look similar to a bar float, but they are shorter and sold in sets of 2 instead of individually like the bar float. Dumbbells provide added resistance in the water during workouts for your arms, shoulders, chest, and back. A water dumbbell is buoyant to increase resistance and ensure you are getting the most out of your workouts. When you exercise with water dumbbells, you can increase the intensity of your workout. Your muscles will work a little harder to perform the same exercise, resulting in more benefits to your overall fitness.

Water dumbbells come in different sizes, so you can choose one that is light, medium or heavy. If you choose multiple sizes, then you can practice with each so you know what you're comfortable with. If you are unsure and do not want multiple sizes, then start with the lightest one and slowly work your way up. Always make sure you can comfortably perform eight reps at a time without too much strain. If you have a variety of different sizes, you can choose an appropriate one for each exercise, and you can steadily increase the weight of the dumbbell you are using as you get more practice.

Most dumbbells are used as part of a set of two, so you can hold one in each hand. There are certain workouts where you will only need one at a time, but it is good practice to purchase them in pairs so you can ensure you're getting an even workout on both sides of your body. Water dumbbells allow you to increase the intensity of a workout while still keeping excessive strain at bay and ensuring your workout remains low impact. They are a key part of any safe and effective exercise plan, so they are worth investing in to perform the workouts in this book.

Other Resistance Equipment

Other resistance equipment is available to you at your own discretion. Visit your local sporting goods store or shop online for other options, some of which are specifically tailored to the pool and some of which can be beneficial in a more general context. For example, you may want to incorporate aqua runners, which are resistance bands that go around your ankles and improve the effectiveness of cardiovascular workouts. Some workouts repurpose swim training gloves, which are large, webbed gloves meant to function like swim paddles, to serve as resistance equipment. Resistance fins around your wrists or ankles can also increase the amount of natural resistance you get just from moving around in the pool. If you check the stores in your area, you may find even more useful tools that can assist you in your workout. Try incorporating a few of them once you have the basics down and you are looking for a little more of a challenge.

CHAPTER 5

What Makes a Workout? Frequency, Steps of a Workout, and Parts of the Body

W hen you think 'workout,' you might only picture the exercises you will be performing. However, a good workout is about much more than just the main exercises. If you were to head to the gym and get right on the treadmill or one of the weight machines, you would quickly find yourself tired and sore. In this scenario, you have not taken the time to limber up, so your muscles and joints are stiff. This limits your range of motion, making it more difficult to use proper form when doing exercises and increasing the amount of soreness you feel afterwards. Additionally, a proper warm-up ensures you are getting good blood flow so the cells in your muscles are receiving the oxygen they need to function. Without one, you will tire out much more quickly. Jumping right into exercises can also increase your risk of injury, so you always want to loosen your body up before you tackle more difficult exercises.

Similarly, it would also be a mistake to complete your exercises and then end your workout, heading home and flopping down on the couch. If you transition very quickly from doing a lot of dynamic and fast-paced movements to being completely still, "your muscles will suddenly stop contracting vigorously. This can cause blood to pool in the lower extremities of your body, leaving your blood without as much pressure to be pumped back to the heart and brain" (Tri-City Medical Center, n.d., para. 16). This can leave you feeling dizzy and can increase your risk of fainting. Therefore, a good cooldown is just as important as a good warm-up.

A complete workout must be as safe and effective as possible for your activity level. The best way to ensure this is to always complete a full workout which includes stretching and warming up as well as a gradual cooldown. Start with a warm-up, move on to your exercises, and then finish with some lower-intensity cooldown exercises to round out the workout. These are the basic foundations of every workout you will do and following this checklist will help you significantly limit your risk of injury.

Of course, while these three steps are the bare bones of a workout, there are many more components you should know and incorporate before you get started. Consider important factors like the frequency of your workouts, how you are going to follow each of the stages, where you want to focus your efforts, flexibility, and other ways you can customize your workout to suit your individual needs.

Frequency

The ideal frequency of a workout depends on what you are trying to achieve with it. People who want to really push themselves may opt to exercise at a high intensity for very long periods of time. On the other hand, if you are just looking to improve your overall health so you can stay in shape and prevent health conditions associated with a lack of exercise, your bar is going to be much lower.

Most experts, such as those at the Department of Health and Human Services, recommend that if you want to keep yourself healthy, you should aim for "150 minutes of moderate aerobic activity or 75 minutes of vigorous aerobic activity a week, or a combination of moderate and vigorous activity" (Laskowski, 2019, para. 2). Of course, you do not need to do all this exercise in one day. In fact, it is much better for your body if you can commit to doing smaller workouts every day or most days. This keeps you from exhausting yourself and ensures that you are staying active on a regular basis, which will provide better benefits than if you restricted exercise to once or twice a week. Working out for as little as 25 minutes three or four times a week can help you comfortably hit your goals.

Remember that, as always, you should be relatively comfortable when working out. If you feel so exhausted you are struggling to keep pace, you are likely pushing yourself too hard. Ease up on your routine and stick to a workout schedule that better suits your capabilities, at least until you build up the muscle and stamina you need to tackle these more intense workouts.

As you continue working out on a routine basis, you will find that each workout will get easier and easier for you to complete. Better yet, you will likely end up making your workouts a bit longer without even noticing it. Even people who are not naturally inclined to exercise often find they enjoy it much more than they initially expected once they have turned exercise into a habit. But in order to stick to a workout plan, you must always consider what frequency you are comfortable with, or you will end up burning all your energy off too quickly.

Increasing Your Intensity

Regular exercise makes it easier to work out for longer periods of time, and it also allows you to push yourself a little harder when you feel ready. If you are up to it, try incorporating higher intensity exercises into your regular workout routines for brief periods of time, cycling between intensities. Start out with a movement at regular intensity. Then perform 30 seconds of the movement at increased intensity, followed by another 30 seconds at regular intensity again. For example, if you are walking in the water, try jogging for 30 seconds before returning to walking again. These short bursts of speed and movement support your cardiovascular health and can help you build muscle and trim fat.

Stages of a Workout

As mentioned earlier in the chapter, workouts come in three stages. These are the warm-up, the exercises, and the cooldown at the end. Each of these three stages are important, so make sure you know how to complete each one for the most effective workout.

Warm-Up

Your warm-up should consist of slow-paced movements and stretches that are meant to increase blood flow, supplying more oxygen to your muscles. It is good practice to do a full body stretch if you have the time, but at the very least, ensure you are stretching the parts of your body that you are about to exercise. If you are going to focus on your legs, do a few leg stretches, such as high knees and hamstring stretches, or whatever you are capable of with your level of mobility. Stretches should not be painful, so if you feel any twinges, relax and ease back until you are stretching only to a comfortable degree.

Remember that your warm-up is the appetizer of your workout, not the main course. There is no sense in warming up until you are exhausted. You want to save all your energy for the actual workouts, so just stretch for a few minutes so you are more limber and ready to go.

Exercises

Start performing exercises as soon as you are done with your warm-ups. It is good to move right into them, as this is the point when you are the most prepared and you have the most energy. Still, you can start with some slightly easier exercises and tackle harder ones when you get into the rhythm.

The exercise portion of your workout should last for at least as long as your warm-up. If you warmed up for ten minutes, shoot for at least ten minutes of good exercise. Still, it is fine if your exercise es are longer than your warm-up. This will naturally occur as you improve your workout stamina over time, so you do not end up with a 25-minute warm-up to accompany your 25-minutes of exercise.

Cooldown

If the warm-up is the appetizer of a workout and the exercises are the main course, then the cooldown is the dessert. However, unlike that chocolate lava cake at the restaurant, your cooldown is actually good for you, and it is mandatory to fully complete the workout. Never skip the cooldown no matter how tired you are, or you will regret it later on. This is because the cooldown helps gradually slow the blood flow throughout your body back to a regular resting level. It also decreases your body temperature, which may be higher than usual after exercising.

Cooldowns should naturally follow the final exercise in your routine without any significant breaks. Make sure your cooldown involves the parts of the body you just exercised. If you worked your arms, shoulders, and chest, your cooldown should involve these muscle groups too. You do not have to do anything fancy for this stage. You can repeat the same stretches and other warm-ups you used at the beginning of the workout, so you will know you are targeting all the relevant muscle groups.

Parts of the Body

While very few individual exercises can affect every muscle in your body, there is an exercise meant to target just about anywhere. If you want to improve your balance by focusing on your legs and torso, you can choose exercises that engage the lower half of your body. If you want to improve your cardiovascular health, you can incorporate higher intensity exercises into your routine. If you prefer to improve your upper arm strength, you can do that too. Ideally, it is a good idea to exercise different areas of your body so no one area falls behind. But whether you are interested in full-body workouts or just accomplishing a specific goal, it helps to know the different muscle groups that various exercises can target.

Focusing Your Workout

Workouts can focus on various zones throughout your body. These include the upper body, lower body, and core, as well as more general workouts that incorporate exercises from each of these areas.

Upper body workouts engage the muscles in your arms, including your wrists and hands. These are ideal if you have arthritis, which can make it harder to bend the joints in your arms, and if you want to build muscle in your bicep area. Upper body workouts also include your shoulders and neck which can frequently feel stiff if you do not take care to keep them moving.

Other workout routines target the muscles in your lower body. These include all of the areas of your legs, from your buttocks, hips, and thighs all the way down to your calves, ankles, and feet. Since your lower body plays a key role in maintaining your balance, as well as contributing to your strength when lifting up heavy objects, these are important muscle groups to involve in your workouts.

Core workouts are centered around engaging the muscles in your mid-section or torso. These include your chest and abdomen, as well as your upper and lower back. Core muscles assist in stabilization, preventing falls and working wonders for your balance. Having a strong core can make it easier for you to complete other kinds of exercises, as it serves as a support system connecting the upper and lower halves of your body. Even if you are not planning on working out until you develop a six-pack, giving your core muscles the attention they need is still crucial.

Some workouts target more than one area of the body. A few routines are specially designed to engage muscles from your upper body, lower body, and core. These are considered full-body or overall body workouts, and they allow you to develop your muscles evenly throughout your body over the course of a single workout. Some days, you may decide to focus on just one area of your body, while others you may prefer to get in a full workout. The important part is that you stay moving and you work to keep yourself as fit as possible.

Other Important Information

Regardless of your personal level of fitness and the intensity of your workout, there are plenty of ways you can customize and improve a given exercise routine. Make sure you are pacing your workout to suit your actual needs and abilities, not the level you think you should be at. Everyone builds muscle at a slightly different rate, and it is okay if you are not capable of tackling more intense workouts, at least not yet. As long as you are staying active, it is okay to adjust your exercise plan to ensure you are getting the most out of it. This means choosing exercises that align with your personal fitness goals, working out for longer or shorter periods, employing rest days effectively, and working with your level of flexibility.

Customizing Your Routine

The benefits of creating your own exercise plan, as opposed to working with a personal trainer or following a rigid routine that has been created for you, is that you can make any customizations you like. If you are having too much trouble keeping up with your workout, slow down and cut out some of the more intense exercises until you are ready for them. If your routine is too easy, feel free to add to it as needed, though take care not to work yourself too hard. If you feel like your workouts are getting a little stale, mix things up and try out new exercises that make you feel more engaged.

You can also customize your workout to focus on helping you achieve the fitness goals you have set for yourself. If you know you struggle with cardio, introduce a few exercises that are performed at a higher intensity to really get your blood pumping. If your main concern is improving flexibility in a stiff limb, make sure your exercises target the area without putting too much strain on it. When you personalize your routine, you set yourself up for future success.

Avoiding Overexertion

Far too many people set unrealistic and unachievable goals for themselves when they start exercising. They look at what other people are doing and decide they must exercise at the same intensity, not realizing that these people have been routinely working out for months or years. If you are starting from scratch, the only thing an hour-long workout is going to do is leave you so exhausted you never want to think about getting back into the pool again.

You can avoid overexertion by starting out with relatively brief workout durations and only moving on when you feel comfortable. It is typically a good idea to start with a workout of no longer than 20-30 minutes. Then divide this time into the different stages of your workout. This gives you about five to eight minutes to warm up. Follow this with 10-15 minutes of exercise. Then take another five to eight minutes to cool down. This will help you determine if this is a good routine length for you or if you're ready for something that is a little more challenging.

Rotating Your Exercises

Engaging different parts of your body in workouts is important, but you do not want to overdo it. It is a good idea to work out the upper body, lower body, and full body separately on different days so you can let yourself rest each area. When you rest up, you ensure that you are ready to tackle your next workout with all your energy and enthusiasm. You will not be held back by your exhausted arms from the previous day if you focus on your legs, and vice versa.

You can even alternate your exercise days and rest days along with the different areas of your body to ensure you are properly recovering in between workouts. For example, in a given week, you might start out by exercising your upper body on Monday, then resting completely on Tuesday. Perform exercises that target the lower body on Wednesday, and rest again on Thursday. This means that when Friday rolls around, both your upper and lower body will be sufficiently well rested, so you can perform an overall body workout that does not put too much strain on your body.

Improving Flexibility

Maintaining a good workout routine will significantly improve your flexibility over time. While age, joint stiffness, and other problems caused by injuries and health conditions can limit your range of movement, becoming more flexible will allow you to regain the use of your muscles and joints slowly over time. Depending on your circumstances, you may not be able to achieve the same range of movement you had in your youth, but you will certainly be able to move much farther and faster with a significantly lower risk of injury.

It is normal to have limited flexibility when you first start out. You might not be able to bend down and touch your toes, or to fully extend your arms to your sides. However, as you continue to work out, your flexibility will improve, and you will be capable of doing many more exercises that were difficult for you originally. Give yourself time to develop your muscles and work your joints and you will be able to accomplish a great deal more than you previously thought possible.

CHAPTER 6

Exercise Program Must-Haves

Your body has different needs depending on your physical condition and where you are in your life. When you are young and healthy, you are generally capable of being more physically active and performing more strenuous activities, but you usually do not need to engage in dedicated exercise nearly as much to keep yourself in shape. Skills like flexibility and balance come more naturally because you are moving around and stretching regularly throughout the day, so you do not always have to make a dedicated effort. Additionally, younger people tend to have fewer issues with joint pain and limited mobility, so when they start working out, they can begin at a higher intensity. They do not have to spend time building these abilities up the same way that you might.

Of course, being older and having mobility issues does not prohibit you from exercising entirely. You just need to work at your own pace and address each area of your health individually. Your workouts should address your balance, flexibility, muscle strength, and cardiovascular health, just like everyone else, but you may need more time to gradually build up these abilities. Maintaining a steady workout routine will allow you to address each of these important areas which all contribute heavily to your overall health and fitness. Begin with balance, then move on to cardiovascular training and strength training when you get the hang of things.

Building a Foundation of Balance

Your balance is the foundation upon which the rest of your exercises will follow. It is incredibly difficult to complete a full workout if you are not able to maintain your balance. You'll find it harder to complete the moves, especially if you are still working on improving your flexibility. You are also running a higher risk of falling over if you cannot keep your balance, which could potentially be dangerous, especially in the pool.

Balance is also an important factor in maintaining good form. Let's say an exercise calls for you to stand up straight and then lift one leg. If this causes you to wobble, you might bend over or reach out, which would put you in a position that might make it more difficult to complete the rest of the exercise. Posture is incredibly important when you are working out, as poor posture increases your risk of injury, especially muscle strain. It also limits the benefits you get from any exercise, as you might not be engaging the right muscles. When you improve your balance, you ensure you can maintain perfect posture as you exercise, so you will not have to worry as much about potential falls and pulled muscles.

When you start working out in the pool, it is a good idea to start with a few balance exercises, even if your balance is usually okay. This will give you a good read on how stable you are and what areas you need to work on so you can properly direct your focus. Remember that in water, your center of balance can be very different from what it is on land. Many people find it easier to maintain their footing in the pool because the water provides buoyancy, while others may be left feeling a little off-balance due to the push and pull of the water. As you get used to the pool and continue to invest time and effort into exercises focused on balance, you will run into fewer issues. From there, you can move on to workouts focused more on flexibility, cardio, and strength, but building that initial level of balance is key.

Creating a Balance Training Routine

Prior to fully developing your sense of balance, you may need some assistance as you work to train yourself. You want to minimize any risk of harm, so it is a good idea to stabilize yourself in the water. You can accomplish this in a few ways. The simplest option is to hold onto the side of the pool as you perform your exercises. Just reach out a hand to hold the edge and perform the exercise to the best of your abilities while minding your proximity to the edge. You can lean some of your weight against the side of the pool, though you should try to use this support as sparingly as possible if you are working to improve your balance.

Another option is to use one of the flotation devices mentioned in Chapter 4. Keeping a hand on a bar float or another device like a noodle can be a huge help. These pieces of equipment provide a little less stability since they float on the water, but this can actually be more beneficial since it allows you to focus more on engaging your core to maintain your balance.

Exercises meant to train your balance do not generally exert your muscles to the same extent as other exercises. They are not going to make you sore or leave you out of breath, so resting in between exercises isn't quite so important here. Therefore, it is okay to do as many balance exercises as you like during a session, since you don't have to worry about exhaustion and recovery. Focus on just your balance for a while before you move on to other kinds of exercises, and even then, it does not hurt to add a balance exercise or two to your warm-up routine. The more practice you get, the easier it will be to complete the rest of your workout.

Training Your Cardiovascular Health

Your cardiovascular health refers to the efficiency at which your heart, lungs, and blood vessels work. Good cardiovascular health is strongly correlated with good overall health and minimizes your risk factors for a variety of different diseases and other health conditions. On the other hand, if you have poor cardiovascular health, this can contribute to bad circulation, plaque buildup in your arteries, high blood pressure, and in some severe cases, heart disease.

Failing to exercise means failing to maintain your cardiovascular health, which can greatly increase your risk of developing multiple health conditions. Heart disease and damage to your blood vessels from years of high blood pressure can lead to complications including peripheral artery disease, heart failure, sudden cardiac arrest, a heart attack, stroke, and an aneurysm (Mayo Clinic Staff, 2021, para. 52). Lung disease and pulmonary embolisms are also common for people with poor cardiovascular health. Many of these complications are life-threatening, so it is critical to be proactive in taking good care of your heart and lungs.

Keep in mind that many factors are at play in determining your risk of cardiovascular problems. Some are out of your control, such as your age and family history. Others are entirely up to you to address to keep yourself as healthy as possible. Eat heart-healthy meals and avoid high-fat and high-sugar diets that raise your blood pressure and increase cholesterol. Find constructive ways of regularly alleviating your stress levels and avoid behaviors that are harming your health like smoking and excessive drinking. And of course, manage your weight and blood pressure through exercise. While exercise may be just one piece in a larger puzzle, it is just as important as any other component. Engaging in even small amounts of heart-healthy exercise each day, just enough to keep you active and address any health concerns, can work wonders for your cardiovascular system. When you work out, you are making an investment in your future.

The Relationship Between Exercise and Cardiovascular Health

Regular use of your heart, lungs, and blood vessels has markedly positive effects on your cardiovascular health. You can accomplish this by making exercise a regular part of your week. Exercises that focus on your stamina are especially beneficial. Even if you are not exactly up to running a mile every morning, you can still practice exercises that involve the same repetitive movement for a prolonged period of time. For example, walking, whether in the pool or on land, engages the same set of muscles and keeps you moving constantly. This works your lungs and helps to keep your blood circulating, reducing the risk of plaque buildup and blockages. The more you are working your heart and lungs, the better off you will be.

Exercise does not have to be particularly strenuous to be effective. Just 30 minutes of moderate-intensity exercises per day can be enough to support your cardiovascular health as long as you are supplementing it with other healthy choices like proper nutrition and getting enough sleep. You can even break these 30-minute sessions up into 10-minute intervals and spread them throughout the day, so you do not overwork yourself at any point. If you are taking a rest day from your workouts, try to incorporate some movement into other parts of your day. This can be as simple as taking the stairs or doing some gardening in the yard; anything that keeps you moving improves circulation and overall cardiovascular health.

If you are worried you will not be able to handle prolonged periods of exercise, you can start out with a less-intense version and work your way up to something more challenging. For example, start out with a slow walk in the pool, and gradually increase your speed. Eventually, you should be able to travel at a brisk pace without issue.

Finally, avoid working so hard that it starts to feel like a struggle to catch your breath. Many people mistakenly believe that a cardio workout is only beneficial if you can feel the burn in your lungs, but in truth, you are only exhausting yourself for little to no benefit. You should be able to hold a conversation while you exercise, so if you are panting heavily enough that it would prevent you from being able to speak, it is time to take a break and tone down the intensity of your exercise. This will allow you to improve your cardiovascular health without engaging in an overwhelming amount of exercise.

Improving Strength with Resistance Training

For resistance training to have a noticeable effect on your muscles, it should be somewhat challenging. You are not going to get much benefit out of performing an easy motion with light weights that provides no resistance at all. At the same time, just like with other kinds of exercise, it is important not to go overboard. Make sure you can still comfortably complete eight reps of any exercise without compromising your form, as too much strain could increase your risk of injury.

If you feel like the exercises are too strenuous for you at first, try them with a lighter weight, or with no weight at all until you build up the relevant muscles. The water provides some resistance on its own, so keep in mind that you may not be able to work out with the amount of weight you think you should be able to handle. Additionally, some exercises are easier than others; a medium-size weight could be completely manageable for one kind of exercise and too strenuous for another. This is why it is always a good idea to buy a few differently sized dumbbells and other resistance equipment, so you can choose one that is the appropriate heaviness for each exercise.

Incorporating Equipment

You can get a more complete workout by using resistance equipment during your workout, especially if the equipment is specifically designed for use in the pool. Many people use water weights, which provide some added resistance against your movements. Using water weights is a great way to increase the intensity of your workout without having to extend the set and rep count or try more challenging exercises.

Water dumbbells are a popular choice because, just like regular dumbbells, they are highly versatile. There are dozens of different exercises that can be performed with just a dumbbell or two. Water dumbbells have the added benefit of being made of foam and plastic, which makes them very lightweight and allows them to float on the surface of the water. If you keep the water dumbbells above the water, you can use them as a handhold to help you maintain your stability during an exercise. Additionally, while you will not experience much resistance if you try to lift them up, attempting to pull or push them down beneath the surface of the water yields much more fruitful results.

You can perform a very simple and easy to learn resistance exercise with just a pair of water dumbbells. Start by holding the dumbbells right on the surface of the water. Then pull them down under the water for a count of three. Hold the dumbbells here for one second, then slowly return them back to the surface, keeping your movements controlled so they last another full three seconds. As a tip, breathe in as you pull the weight down, and breathe out as you slowly return to the starting position. Do not forget to rest between reps if you feel you need a short break before trying the exercise again.

Other kinds of water resistance equipment can improve the effectiveness of your workout as well. Typically, you should only add additional resistance once your balance, endurance, and stamina has improved, so wait until you have been exercising in the pool for long enough to feel comfortable and confident in the water. Check online listings and local fitness stores to see what is available near you. Plenty of water resistance equipment is specially designed to help you target specific body parts. They may include weights or fins that increase resistance for your arms and legs. There are tools you can attach to your hands or wrists, hold in your hands, put on your legs, and put on your feet. Make sure to coordinate these tools with the kind of workout you are doing. If you are focusing on your lower body, use resistance weights for your legs or feet. If it is a rest day for your lower body, try equipment that targets your upper body instead. You get to control what part of your body you are working out each day based on your exercise program. Just remember to keep your workout even and schedule some rest days, and you will have a great routine that provides a decent challenge without being too strenuous.

CHAPTER 7

Balance Exercises

B alance exercises target your lower body. They often focus on moving each leg separately, which helps you practice supporting yourself with just one leg on the bottom of the pool. These exercises also improve your ability to shift your center of balance from one side of your body to the other. Remember to engage your core muscles as you work through each of these exercises, as this will help you maintain your balance. You can also keep a hand on the side of the pool or a flotation device to hold yourself steady before you have fully built up your balance.

It is vital to have a strong sense of balance before attempting any other kinds of exercises in the pool, so start with these and work your way up to more challenging movements. A few quick balance exercises at the beginning of every workout can help you find your footing in the pool even as you continue to improve your skills.

Balance on One Leg

Balancing on one leg is a very simple exercise, but it is great for improving your stability. If you find yourself leaning to one side, remember to tighten your core muscles. You can also try focusing on a static point a few feet in front of you.

Lift right foot

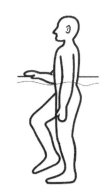

1. Start with both feet planted firmly on the bottom of the pool. Lift your right foot off the ground and shifting your center of balance to your left foot.

2. Hold your foot in the air for a few seconds, depending on how long you can remain steady in this position. You can start with a five second hold and increase the amount of time you spend balancing on one leg to about 20-30 seconds as you improve.

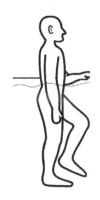

3. Gradually lower your right foot back down to the pool floor.

Lift left foot

4. Bend and lift your left foot, balancing on your right foot. Hold this position for a few seconds.

5. Return your left foot to the ground slowly.

6. Repeat the exercise for as many reps as desired, alternating your feet each time.

Balance on One Leg with Arm Lifted

When you feel stable enough to balance on one leg fairly comfortably, you can switch to a slightly more challenging exercise. When you lift your arm during this exercise, you slightly shift your center of gravity. This will help you build up your sense of balance for future exercises, as you are getting yourself used to moving while maintaining that same steady core.

1. From a relaxed standing position, raise your left arm into the air. Try to hold it straight up over your head or as close to straight as you can comfortably go.

2. Without letting your arm drop back down, lift your left leg and shift your weight to balance on your right foot.

3. Hold this position for 10 seconds, breathing deeply and tightening your core muscles if you start to feel wobbly.

4. Slowly return your foot to the floor and your arm to your side. Then repeat the exercise with your right arm and leg.

5. Continue performing reps until you complete a full set, alternating the left and right sides of your body.

Weight Transfer from One Leg to the Other

Learning how to shift your weight smoothly and safely in the pool will help you remain stable while performing all kinds of exercises. This skill can also benefit you in your daily life as well, reducing the likelihood of falls and related injuries.

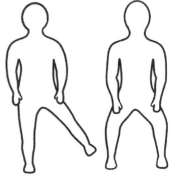

1. Spread your feet shoulder-width apart, bending your knees slightly to lower your center of gravity.

2. Slowly lean over to the right, keeping your right foot firmly on the ground and shifting your weight over. As you lean, lift your left leg up a few inches so it is hovering above the ground.

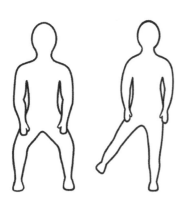

3. Hold this pose for 30 seconds. If you cannot manage the whole 30 seconds, start with shorter reps and gradually build up your tolerance through practice.

4. Return your left foot back to the ground, then resettle your weight so it is evenly distributed between both feet.

5. Next, repeat the process but on your left side. Lean your weight onto your left foot while raising your right foot above the ground.

6. Again, hold the pose for 30 seconds or as long as you can comfortably manage.

7. Return your right foot to the ground and recenter your weight once again.

8. Continue repeating the exercise, alternating your feet each time.

Leg Kicks

Leg kicks are a great way to work the muscles in your lower body. They target the glutes, quads, and hamstrings, giving you more power in your legs and a greater sense of stability as you move through the water. Better yet, they are a very versatile exercise, so you can target different muscle areas and shake up your workout to prevent strain.

Sideways Leg Kicks

During sideways leg kicks, you swing your leg out to the side of your body, then repeat the motion with the opposite leg. This works your glutes while also improving mobility in your hip joint, which broadens your range of motion.

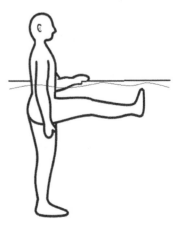

1. Shift your weight to your left leg. Hold on to the edge of the pool or a flotation device on your left side, if you need to.

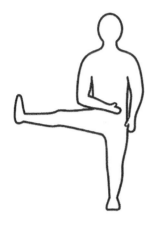

2.   Lift your right leg in the water directly out in front of you. Try to keep your leg straight and parallel to the surface of the water, if possible.

3.   While maintaining your balance on your left leg, swing your right leg out to the side in one fluid movement. Go as far as you can but stop if you experience any pain or discomfort. Your range of motion will improve with practice, making this part of the exercise easier over time.

4. Bring your leg back in front of your body without bending it. Then let your foot return to the base of the pool, coming to rest in a relaxed position.

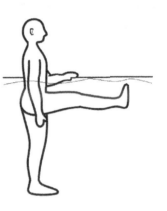

Repeat the exercise, this time keeping your weight on your right foot and kicking your left leg out.

Sideways Leg Kicks with One Arm

If you want to work your upper and lower body at the same time, incorporate some arm movements into the standard leg kick exercise. Make sure you can keep your balance without the support of holding onto the edge of the pool before attempting this exercise. To perform a sideways leg kick with one arm raised, follow the same steps as the previous exercise with these additions.

1. As you lift your right leg in front of you, mimic the motion with your right arm, raising it straight out in front of you as well.

2. When you swing your leg to the right, swing your arm to the right as well. When you are bringing your leg back to the starting position at the end of the rep, do the same with your arm.

3. Repeat the same process with your left arm and leg, alternating the side of your body you are engaging.

4. If you want some added resistance, try performing this exercise in chest-deep water. This way, your arms remain underwater, and you get to enjoy the additional benefits created by pushing against the water tension as you work out.

Forward and Backward

Forward and backward leg movements are another great way to become more flexible and balanced. The joint in your hip bone is known as a ball-and-socket joint, which is why you can rotate your leg in so many directions. This means that if you want to make your range of motion as wide as possible, you need to include both forward and backward movements with side-to-side exercises.

1. Start in a loose, comfortable stance. Make sure you are standing so you have plenty of space in front of you and behind you. You can reach to your side to hold the edge of the pool. Then shift your weight to your left leg.

2. Raise your right leg up and point it straight out in front of you. Lift it as far forward as you can comfortably move and hold this leg extension for a beat.

3. Maintaining a steady pace, swing your leg under and then behind you, going as far back as you can comfortably move once again. This may be a bit more difficult than kicking your leg forward since it is a less common motion in everyday activities, but with some practice you should be able to extend your leg behind you fairly far.

4. Bring your leg back into the resting position. Then shift your center of balance to the right side of your body and repeat the exercise with your left leg.

Forward and Backward with One Arm

Just like the sideways leg kicks, you can incorporate arm movements into this exercise as well. Just like the joint in your hips, there are ball-and-socket joints in your shoulders as well, and it is just as necessary to exercise with the full range of motion in your upper body as it is to do so in your lower body. This works wonders for your balance and helps to ensure you are getting an even workout. To add in arm movements, perform the same exercise as described above but with a few additions.

1. When you swing your right leg forward, move your left arm forward as well. It is more helpful to use the arm opposite from the leg you're moving for this exercise, as this will keep you steady and limit the risk of overbalancing.

2. When you swing your right leg down and back behind you, repeat the same motion with your left arm.

3. When you move your left leg forward and back, mimic these motions with your right arm as well.

Forward Lean

The forward lean is a great way to improve your ability to shift your weight, which will help you keep your movements fluid in future exercises, reducing the risk of injury. During this exercise, you will move from a relaxed position to balancing on the balls of your feet, holding yourself up with your arms. This allows you to ease into the new position carefully and safely.

1. Begin the exercise facing the side of the pool. Step back far enough that you can almost fully extend your arms in front of you without brushing the pool's edge, but not so far that you cannot get a firm grip on it without bending forward.

2. While holding the edge of the pool, bring your feet together, and keep your back and legs in a straight vertical line.

3. Gradually lean forward toward the pool's edge, making sure your grip is secure and you are not at risk of slipping. Maintain the straight line of your legs and back. As you move, lift up the back of your feet a little so you are putting your weight on the balls of your feet and bending your toes.

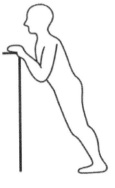

4. Hold this position for a moment. If you feel yourself starting to get a little wobbly, you can break the pose early so you are not at risk of falling and injuring yourself.

5. Slowly straighten your arms to push yourself back into the standing position that is the starting position.

These balance exercises represent the very tip of the iceberg of your exercise journey. They are meant to prepare you for the challenges you will face with future exercises. Remember that you can always use a few balance exercises before you start a more intense workout. At the same time, they are far from the only low-intensity exercises that help to warm up and cool down your muscles, so make sure to mix it up and always target the muscles and joints you will be using in the rest of your workout.

CHAPTER 8

Warm-Up and Cooldown Exercises

The warm-up is one of the most important parts of your workout routine, so it is key to take care to get it right. At the same time, there are many different options available to you which may be appropriate for different kinds of workouts and fitness levels. Picking the right warm-ups will allow you to exercise without fear of injury while also improving the effectiveness of every exercise you perform. The cooldown period at the end of your workout is equally important, as it bridges the gap between exercise and resting in a way that alleviates muscle strain and improves the benefits of the workout.

This chapter lists many different warm-up and cooldown exercises, so do not feel like you have to include them all for every workout. In fact, if you were to perform all of these exercises, you would only succeed in exhausting yourself and putting too much strain on your body. Instead, pick and choose the ones that are relevant to the muscles you will be exercising, as well as those that work best for your individual body, muscles, and joints. Additionally, try rotating your warm-up and cooldown selections so you are never overtaxing any one muscle group. Relying too heavily on the same warm-ups or doing too many warm-ups often leads to soreness and joint stiffness, which can be just as harmful as not warming up or cooling down at all.

When selecting what warm-ups and cooldowns you want to do, remember to consider your own abilities and limitations. Everyone has limits, and while these limits can be gradually expanded through repeated exercise, it is not fair to expect yourself to be able to handle everything right away, nor is it safe. Read through all of the options first before you decide which ones might work best for you. You should avoid any movements that aggravate especially stiff or injured muscles, joints, or appendages unless you are working with a trained physical therapist. If something gives you trouble or pain when you move it, it is best to avoid unnecessary strain. If you can perform an exercise once or twice but only with great difficulty, then do not repeat it, and instead select something else. Always maintain your comfort while working out even as you push yourself.

The warm-up and cooldown exercises in this chapter are divided into sections based on the muscle groups that are worked. These are the upper body, lower body, and core body.

Upper Body

Perform upper body warm-ups and cooldowns on days when you plan on exercising your upper body muscles, such as those in your shoulders, arms, neck, and upper back. You have many smaller muscles in these areas which may be heavily strained if you do not take time to get them moving before doing any heavy lifting.

Finger Walk

When you think about exercise, working out your fingers may not be the first thing that comes to mind, but the muscles and joints here are just as important to keep moving as more noticeable muscle groups. The finger walk can help reduce swelling, inflammation, and pain from arthritis and other joint conditions. It will also improve your ability to hold onto the edge of the pool, a water dumbbell, or a flotation device without your fingers feeling sore and cramped.

1. Sit down on the steps in the pool. you can also kneel in the shallow end as long as your head is still comfortably above the water. Your hands should be submerged.

2. Extend, stretch, and wiggle your fingers while letting them rest on the pool's step, edge or even on your leg.

3. Move your fingers in a spider walk across your chosen surface, making sure to keep your entire hand underwater. You want the gentle resistance of the water to push back against your fingers as you perform this exercise.

4. Finger walk with each hand, taking care to stretch all of the muscles and joints as you do so.

Wrist Rolls

The wrists are a common site of injury during exercise, in part because many people forget they should be addressed during a warm-up. These wrist rolls allow you to do exactly that, drastically reducing the likelihood that you will pull or sprain a muscle in your forearms during your workout.

1. Hold your arms out in front of you so they are near each other.

2. Bend your arms at the elbow.

3. Clasp your hands together with your fingers entwined loosely.

4. Begin in a circular motion to the right, in a figure-eight

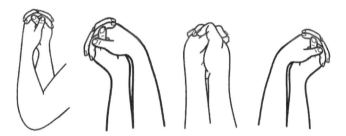

or semi-circle motion.

Boxer Punches

Boxer punches engage both your forearms and your upper arms, as well as parts of your shoulders and upper back. They are a great way to round out your warm-up or cooldown. As the name implies, you will be moving your arms in a punching motion with your fists clenched, which naturally stretches these muscles.

1. If you are comfortable being in a depth of water that just covers your shoulders, then do so for this warm-up. You can also sit or kneel in the shallow end to allow the water to cover your arms and shoulders.

2. Curl your fingers into loose fists. Then, take up a boxing stance. This means bending your elbows, so your fists are raised up near your chin.

3. Punch forward with your right fist, then return to your starting position. Keep your movement slow and fluid while punching straight out rather than curving as you might if you were hitting a training bag. Your goal is to stretch your muscles out, not to actually strike an object with any real force. You should be punching out in front of you.

4. Repeat the same motion with your left fist.

5. Continue alternating punches. Use minimal force, as you are just trying to get the blood flowing in your muscles.

Shoulder and Upper Arm Stretch

A good stretch loosens up the tension in your muscles and allows you to move more freely as you exercise. Stretching your shoulders and upper arms is a great way to prepare for more intense upper body workouts, especially those that require a wider range of motion to complete with good form.

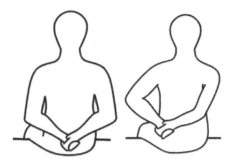

1. Sit down on the steps in the pool. Bring your arms behind your back, then clasp your hands together near the base of your spine.

2. Slowly swing your clasped hands to the left, stretching out your right shoulder and upper arm. You can gently twist your trunk to deepen the stretch as well.

3. Bring your hands back to the center behind your back, then swing them to the right. Stretch your left shoulder and upper arm.

4. Repeat this exercise several times on both sides until your arm muscles feel sufficiently loosened.

Upper Arm Stretch

The upper arms stretch targets the backs of your upper arms with a gentle pulling motion. You can alter the exercise in a few ways to adjust the level of stretch you get.

1. Raise your right arm up in the air. Turn your palm so it faces in toward your body.

2. Bend your elbow and position your arm so your hand falls behind your head. Your elbow should point straight up in the air next to your right ear.

3. Hold this position to stretch the back of the upper arm.

4. Return to the starting pose, then repeat these movements with your left arm as well. Continue alternating your arms to deepen the stretch.

Achieve an even more extensive stretch by performing the following additions if you feel you are capable of them without causing discomfort.

1. Follow the above directions so your right arm is bent and your hand is behind your head.

2. Bring your left arm up into the air above you.

3. Bend your left elbow, reaching over and gently grasping your right elbow.

4. While maintaining your grip, lean your left arm out to the side, gently pulling your right arm.

5. If you would like to go even deeper, try leaning your head and arms a little to the left while holding this pose. From here, you can release your left hand and put your both arms down to return to a neutral position.

Lower Arm Stretch

If you are planning an exercise routine that works your arms, do not forget to target your forearms in your warm-up and cooldown. Show your lower arms some attention with this stretch that also targets your wrists and the joints in your elbows.

1. Stand so you are facing the edge of the pool. Hold your arms out in front of you loosely.

2. Extend your right arm so your palm lies flat against the side of the pool wall. Keep your fingers pointed upward.

3. Lift your right hand away from the wall a little, rotating it clockwise by a few degrees. Return your hand to the pool wall.

4. Repeat this motion a few times, turning your hand a little further with each rep. Remember that you should only go as far as is comfortable for you.

5. Once you have turned your hand as far as possible

without discomfort at your current level of flexibility, start rotating the same hand counterclockwise to return to the starting position.

6. Repeat these steps with your left arm for an even warm-up.

Rolling Your Shoulders

There is nothing like a good shoulder roll to alleviate tension in your upper back. Here are the best steps that will create the most effective stretch before and after your workouts.

1. Start with your arms held comfortably at your sides. Then shrug your shoulders, lifting them straight up and holding in this position to begin the exercise.

2. Roll your shoulders forward and down, moving them in as wide of a semi-circle as you can on your way back to a natural pose.

3. Next, roll your shoulders back behind your body and upward, bringing your shoulders up as high as possible.

4. Repeat these steps but move through them backward. Drop your shoulders back and down first, then roll them forward and up.

5. Repeat until you feel loose and ready to move.

Lean and Stand

The lean and stand exercise stretches out your calves and arms at the same time, which makes it a good choice for upper body workouts that also incorporate some lower body movements. Note that this warm-up can be more difficult if you struggle to support yourself with your arms, so always try it out at a low speed and rep count before deciding whether or not it should be part of your warm-up and cooldown routines.

1. Stand so you are facing the edge of the pool. Reach out and hold the pool's edge, standing far enough away that your arms are nearly straight. Get a firm grip on the lip of the pool before proceeding.

2. Plant your feet shoulder-width apart, adopting a firmly rooted stance.

3. While keeping your feet flat on the bottom of the pool, slowly lean forward, carefully controlling the speed of your lean with your arm muscles. You should feel a gentle pulling sensation in your calves, but if it becomes uncomfortable, you may need to get closer to the pool's edge.

4. Once you have leaned forward, hold this pose for a moment, then push yourself back to an upright position with your arm muscles.

5. Repeat the exercise as needed.

Lower Body

Your lower body is responsible for balance and a great deal of your strength, which means you should never skip out on your warm-ups and cooldowns on leg days. Get a good stretch from your hips down to your toes before you start working these muscles.

Toe Point

The toe point targets the lower leg and foot area, especially the calves and the arches of your feet. This improves your ability to bend and lean while maintaining a stable stance.

1. Sit down on the steps of the pool, then straighten your legs out in front of you.

2. Point your feet and toes forward as far as they can go. Hold this pose, getting a deep stretch that you should be able to feel through your shins and into your legs.

3. Resting your heels on the step, rotate your feet back toward your body, flexing and pointing your toes so they curve toward your torso. Again, hold this position for a few beats.

4. Repeat the exercise a few times to fully loosen your muscles.

Lunge

The lunge is a classic warm-up exercise that is great for getting the blood moving in your legs. It is especially useful for stretching out your upper thighs, so you may also want to perform this exercise when you have been sitting in the same position for a while to prevent soreness and stiffness.

1. Stand with one leg about a foot or more in front of the other. You should be able to lean forward slightly without losing your balance, but do not hold your feet so far apart that the pose is uncomfortable.

2. Straighten your back. You should also keep the leg of the rear foot straight throughout the exercise.

3. Keeping both feet flat on the ground, slowly bend the front knee and lower yourself down into the lunge. If you feel off-balance, you can stand back up

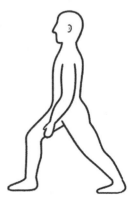

and reposition your feet until you find a comfortable distance.

4. Hold the lunge for about 30 seconds, or a little less if you cannot keep yourself stable the whole time.

5. Straighten your front leg until you are back to the starting stance. Switch the position of your feet, then repeat the exercise.

Knee Lift

Do not forget to stretch the backs of your legs if you are going to perform higher intensity exercises. These knee lifts target the backs of your thighs, specifically your hamstring muscles, and the glute muscles in your buttocks.

1. Start by holding onto the edge of the pool with your left hand. When you have built up your balance, you can let go of the edge, but the extra support is helpful as you find your footing.

2. Lift your left leg up in front of you, bending it at the knee.

3. Place your right hand on the raised knee, then gently pull it toward your chest. Only pull your leg as far as is comfortable for you.

4. Hold this pose for a few moments, ensuring you get the full benefits of the stretch.

5. Lower your leg back to the floor of the pool.

6. Switch hands so you are holding onto the pool's edge with your right hand. Then repeat the exercise with your right leg.

Hip Swing

If you struggle with mobility, stretching out your hip joints can be a big help. This hip swing move gently works the muscles in this area to help you achieve a wider range of motion.

1. Face the pool's edge and hold onto it with your right hand.

2. Shift your weight so your center of balance is on your right side.

3. In essence, you will be swinging one leg at a time from one side of your body to the other during this warm - up.

4. Lift your left foot forward just a few inches, then swing it out to the left side of your body. See how far you can stretch your leg without discomfort.

5. Following a semi-circle path, swing your left leg back down to the starting position and continue with the motion over to your right side so it crosses over your right leg. Be careful not to bump the edge of the pool with your toes. Avoid rotating your hips for the best warm-up.

6. Arc your left leg back to the left side of your body, then repeat this motion several times with the same leg.

7. When you have finished with the left leg, let go of the edge with your right hand, turn your body to face the other direction and grab it with your left hand instead.

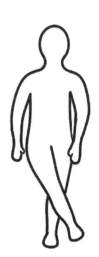

8. Repeat the exercise, this time swinging your right leg from side to side.

9. You can add a little extra challenge to this exercise through the use of a pool noodle. Tie the noodle into a knot, then slip your foot into the knot. As you perform the exercise, the noodle will create added resistance.

Front of the Thigh Stretch

The quadriceps, also known as the quads, are located in the front of the thigh. These muscles help you bend and straighten your legs. They are some of the strongest muscles in your body, so it's important to exercise them regularly. That means giving them a proper warm-up and cooldown treatment.

1. Hold the edge of the pool with your left hand and put your weight on your left leg.

2. Bend your right knee and raise your leg behind you. Your foot should be as close to your buttocks as possible.

3. If your foot is near the right side of your buttocks, grab onto it with your right hand. Take a moment to stabilize yourself if you feel a little wobbly.

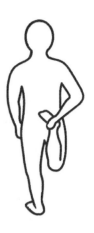

4. If your foot is near the left side of your buttocks instead, you will have trouble stretching your thighs from this position. Start the exercise over, but this time turn yourself, so you are holding the edge of the pool with your right hand. This allows you to reach down and grab your raised foot with your left hand instead.

5. If you can pull your foot a little closer to your glutes, do so. Then hold this position for a few moments.

6. Let go of your foot and slowly bring it back down to the base of the pool. Then repeat the exercise with your other leg to stretch out both sets of quads.

Squats

Squats are a tried-and-true exercise that offer a great way to strengthen the muscles in your lower body. They are especially useful for warming up and cooling down before and after you engage in exercises that target your glutes.

1. Stand with your feet shoulder-width apart. You can hold onto the edge of the pool or a flotation device if you feel like you need the extra stability.

2. While keeping your back straight, bend both knees to squat down. Avoid sticking your hips back any further than they need to go.

3. In one slow, fluid motion, straighten your legs and stand back up. One of the most important tips when performing a squat is to go slow and steady. Quick, jerky movement can increase tension in your knees and cause soreness.

4. Repeat the previous steps until you feel sufficiently warmed up or cooled down.

High Kicks

If your mobility is limited, you may struggle to lift your legs up into the air. These high kicks can help you warm up for any exercise that involves these kinds of leg movements. With practice, you can greatly improve your ability to comfortably move through the motions.

1. Hold onto the edge of the pool if you need it. If you would prefer to have a little more space while still maintaining your stability, use a flotation device for added support, or lean your back against the edge of the pool and grab onto it with your arms stretched out to each side.

2. Keep both of your legs straight as you kick one leg forward and upward. Lift your leg as high as you can.

Ideally, you want to get your leg parallel to the surface of the water.

3. Lower your leg, moving slow and steady rather than releasing all the tension in your muscles at once.

4. Repeat the same kick with the opposite leg. Keep in mind that you may be able to go higher with one leg than you can with the other, so do not push yourself too hard if you notice your kicks are a little uneven.

5. To give an added stretch to your hip, kick your right leg a little to the left, instead of just straight forward.

6. To give this exercise some added challenge, tie a knot in a pool noodle and slip your foot into the center of the knot. The noodle will act as added resistance as you perform the exercise.

Core Body

Your core, which is primarily made up of your abdominal muscles, is heavily involved in exercises that train your balance. It also allows you to twist your torso, and a strong core ensures you are always supporting the upper and lower halves of your body. Even if you are not looking to develop a six-pack, be sure to perform warm-ups and exercises that target your core frequently, as this will make the rest of your workout much easier.

Core Rotations

Core rotations, also known as standing trunk twists, work your abs and obliques. They are a great first step for conditioning your core, as they help to build up the muscles that allow you to bend at the waist and rotate in either direction. These muscles are engaged in a number of different exercises, so spending a little time performing core rotations at the beginning and end of your workouts will be well worth the effort.

1. Place your feet shoulder-width apart. Let them rest flat on the bottom of the pool and avoid lifting up on the balls of your feet throughout the exercise.

2. Turn your head toward the right and allow your shoulders to follow the movement. As you turn, breathe in deeply. Keep turning far enough that you twist your torso to the right and hold this pose for a moment.

3. Turn back to the left so you are looking straight ahead, also straightening out your shoulders and torso. Breathe out as you return to the starting position.

4. Breathing in once again, look to the left this time, twisting your shoulders and core to follow suit.

5. Release your breath as you turn back toward the center.

6. Repeat as necessary, always making sure you are turning far enough that your stomach and chest are engaged in the movement.

Arm Reaches

It is important to stretch your core muscles vertically alongside the horizontal stretch you get from core rotations.

This exercise engages your arms, but it primarily targets the muscles in your abdominal region. You can try this stretch the easy way, as described in the first few steps, or increase the difficulty and effectiveness by adding the modifier mentioned at the end of the directions.

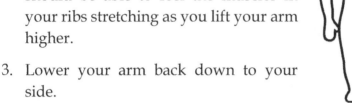

1. Stand in the pool with your feet shoulder-width apart.

2. Take your right hand and stretch it up above your head. Straighten your arm and reach as high up as you can go. You should be able to feel the muscles in your ribs stretching as you lift your arm higher.

3. Lower your arm back down to your side.

4. Repeat the same motion with your left arm, reaching up and then bringing it back to the starting position.

5. If you want to get an even deeper stretch, incorporate leaning to the side, which targets the obliques on either side of your body. When you have your right hand in the air, lean your torso to the left so your right arm is over your head, and when you raise your left hand, lean your torso to the right so your left arms is over your head.

6. Perform this stretch multiple times. Try to reach up a little further each time you repeat it.

Chest Stretch

The chest stretch targets not only your core, but also your shoulder and back muscles. It is a great all-over exercise that emphasizes the importance of a good core warm-up and cooldown when exercising.

1. Stand in the deep end of the pool. The water should come up to your shoulders. Keep your feet about shoulder-width apart, which helps stabilize you while in deeper waters.

2. Reach your arms in front of you with your hands close together moving your arms forward with your shoulders and not your hips. With this you should feel the stretch throughout your upper arms and back.

3. Move your arms away from each other and out to your sides, then behind your back. Go as far behind yourself as is comfortable so you can feel the stretch across your chest. Your arms will not be parallel to the surface but angled downward behind you.

4. Slowly bring your arms back to the starting position and repeat the exercise to continue stretching out your back and chest.

Good warm-ups and cooldowns enable you to really get the most out of every workout. They are important for making sure you are safe both in the pool and out of it. Do not skimp on these exercises in favor of the more challenging ones, or you will experience greater soreness and you will not be nearly loosened up enough to enjoy the benefits of your other exercises. When you focus on getting your blood moving and your muscles pumping in your upper body, lower body, and core, you prepare yourself physically and mentally for the challenges that are to come, so you can face them and overcome them. From here, you can focus on more intense exercises, like cardiovascular workouts and strength training.

CHAPTER 9

Cardiovascular Exercises

I t can be difficult to find good cardiovascular exercises that are effective for you without being outside of your capabilities. If you have an injury that is holding you back or if you are not as young as you used to be, you may not be able to address your cardiovascular health concerns by hitting the treadmill or doing jumping jacks. These kinds of exercises are high-impact, and the jostling of your bones and joints can be very harmful. There is a good chance you will injure yourself if you are not careful, and exercise should never cause you harm. At the same time, if you fail to take care of your heart and lung health and you remain stagnant all day, your overall wellbeing will decline. Therefore, it is important to find a cardiovascular workout routine that suits your needs without being too intense.

The exercises in this chapter are meant to get you moving in a way that should not be too strenuous for you. While everyone's physical limits are a little different, these exercises are designed to be easy on the joints, so there is little risk of injury or overexertion. You can also modify your cardio workout as needed to prioritize less strenuous workouts or shorten the length of your workout to keep yourself from tiring out. Consider interspersing cardio exercises with ones that support balance or strength to round out your workout and reduce the risk of exhaustion. As long as you are paying attention to how you feel as you work out and taking breaks as necessary, you should have no trouble incorporating cardio into your regular exercise routines.

Marching

Marching on land can cause discomfort if you have issues with joint pain. It can be hard to raise your leg up all the way, and the contact of your foot against hard pavement is jarring. When you start marching in the water, however, many of these concerns become non-issues. Moving around is easier on your joints in the water, and the added tension from the water ensures you are not moving too fast as you bring your foot back down. Additionally, the water adds resistance, which increases the effectiveness of the exercise without over-straining your muscles.

1. Stand parallel to the edge of the pool. Reach out and stabilize yourself with a hand on the pool wall if you need to.

2. Marching is similar to walking, but you lift your knees up high with each step. When you raise your leg, it should be bent at the knee at a 90-degree angle, similar to how it would look if you were sitting. However, if raising your leg up high and bending it this far causes some discomfort, it is okay to take it easy until you've started to build up your muscles.

3. If you are holding the pool's edge, march in place, alternating legs with every step.

4. If you feel comfortable enough that you do not have to hold the edge of the pool, you can march around the outside, or just in the shallow end if the pool gets deeper. You should be able to stand with your head and shoulders above the water at all times when performing this exercise, so only go as deep as is comfortable.

5. While you do not want to submerge yourself, you can head to the deep end of the pool if you are ready to make the exercise a little more challenging. Move deep enough that your arms are submerged and swing them as you march. Keeping them underwater ensures the exercise remains low impact while also creating additional resistance that helps to work the upper and lower halves of your body at the same time.

Walking

Walking is one of the simplest possible exercises, but that does not mean it is ineffective. In fact, when you take this everyday activity into the pool, you can greatly increase its benefits thanks to the added water tension. Walking in the cool water is a great way to soothe inflamed and swollen joints as well, which lets you work out harder and for a longer period of time.

1. Hold on to the edge of the pool if you need to.

2. Walk regularly just like you would when you are on land. Preferably, you should be able to walk straight

across the pool, but this may be difficult in pools that get deeper the further you go. If you do not feel comfortable letting go of the edge to walk from one wall to the other instead, you can walk around the edge and simply turn around when the water gets too deep for comfortable movement.

3. Make sure not to walk on your toes, as this interferes with the workout and creates a higher risk of slipping. As you take each step, place your heel down first, then roll your weight onto the bottom of your foot. Then you can safely transfer your weight from the ball of your foot to your toes.

4. If you feel comfortable enough with this exercise and you can walk in the deeper areas of the pool, you can modify this exercise similarly to the changes made to marching for an added challenge. Keep your arms underwater to minimize the impact on your joints and swing them continuously as you walk.

Jogging

When you are ready for something a little more intense than walking, you can try jogging in the pool. Remember that this does not mean you have to exhaust yourself by running as fast as you can. Instead, set a slow, easy pace you can maintain for a few minutes, which will be easy on your joints, heart, and lungs.

1. Hold onto the edge of the pool if you need to.

2. Jog just like you would on land. Head across the pool to the other side if you do not need to grab the edge for

support, as this ensures you will be at the same water depth for the duration of the exercise.

3. If you are holding onto the edge, only go as far as is comfortable for you. When it gets too deep to jog or stand, you can simply turn around and head back the way you came.

4. Jog at an even, enjoyable pace. You should move faster than if you were just walking, which will increase your heart rate, but slower than a full-on run to prevent exhaustion.

5. If you are comfortable in the deep end and you want to make the exercise more challenging, swing your arms as you jog while keeping them underwater.

Bunny Hop

Do not worry if you are not capable of jumping while on land. When you are in the pool, the buoyancy of the water makes it easier to lift off the ground, and the impact of landing back on the floor is not nearly so jarring. This makes the pool the perfect place to perform bunny hop exercises if you are looking to minimize your risk of injury.

1. Stand up straight and hold the edge of the pool. You can perform bunny hops away from the edge once you have tried them out a few times, but it is a good idea to stabilize yourself when you are starting out as this allows you to catch yourself if you slip.

2. Bend your knees a little, then straighten them. Keep your feet flat on the bottom of the pool as you repeat

this motion a few times. This helps to warm up your joints in preparation for the jump.

3. Once you feel comfortable, you can hop off the ground a few inches when you straighten up. Propel yourself forward as you jump so you are moving slowly and steadily along the edge of the pool.

4. Keep hopping, but only go as deep as you feel comfortable. When the water comes up to your shoulders or neck, turn around, grab the edge of the pool with your other hand (if needed), and hop back the way you came.

5. If you want to mix it up and give yourself a challenge, try alternating legs. Hop on one foot two or three times in a row, then switch to the other foot. This is a great exercise for improving your balance as well.

Swim With a Kickboard

If you are a little uncertain about your swimming skills, especially when it comes to maintaining the stamina required to keep yourself afloat, try swimming with a kickboard. The kickboard floats in the water, allowing you to rest your upper body on the board and target the muscles in your core and legs. You can then propel yourself through the water, and if you start to feel tired while in the deep end, you have the board for support as you swim back over to the shallow end of the pool.

1. Take a kickboard into the pool and hold it out in front of you. Grab the board firmly on both sides and lean forward over it so your upper body feels supported.

2. Stretch your legs out behind you and kick your feet to swim from one end of the pool to the other. When you reach the wall, turn around and come back, then repeat the exercise for as many reps as you like.

3. While this exercise is best performed with a kickboard, you can also practice stationary swimming without one. Stretch your arms out in front of you and hold onto the edge of the pool instead. Then lift yourself up so you are floating along the surface on your stomach. Kick your legs like you would while swimming to increase your heart rate.

Swimming

No set of pool exercises would be complete without swimming. Swimming is an excellent way to get your heart rate up and work your muscles at the same time. Professional swimmers are some of the fittest athletes, and while you might not exactly be headed to the Olympics anytime soon, you can still incorporate swimming into your workout routine for phenomenal results.

Rather than following a detailed list of specific steps, you can treat swimming like a leisure activity and approach it however you like. There is no wrong way to swim as long as you are keeping yourself afloat and you are not overworking yourself. Choose any style you are most comfortable with and perform as many laps as you feel are necessary for a complete workout. Whether you are more familiar with the doggy paddle than the breaststroke or butterfly, it is fine to swim however you like. There is no maximum age limit for swimming, and you can be as relaxed or as refined as you prefer.

Your cardiovascular health is incredibly important. A healthy heart and healthy lungs are key to living a long and happy life, so do not skimp on these exercises even if they feel more difficult than non-aerobic ones. Your body will thank you for all your hard work, and the rewards will be well worth the trouble.

CHAPTER 10

Strengthening Exercises

When you think 'exercise,' there is a good chance your mind conjures up a picture of a typical strength workout complete with dumbbells. This is not without a good reason, as strength training is another very important way to improve your physical health and reduce the aches and pains caused by arthritis, age, and many health conditions. On top of this, exercises that focus on helping you build muscle mass also assist in improving your physique, as they are one of the most effective ways of toning various areas of the body. Therefore, strength exercises help you both look and feel good, and their benefits speak for themselves.

Strength exercises are also commonly referred to as resistance training because they involve the use of weights and other resistance equipment to put a healthy amount of tension on your muscles. This tension leads to muscle growth, but this increase in muscle mass is just one of the many positive effects of this type of exercise. When you perform resistance exercises on a regular basis, you will also notice you feel stronger, and you will have less trouble handling everyday tests of your strength. You might find that you can make one less trip when bringing the groceries in from the car, or that you have more stamina when going for a walk. Additionally, resistance training can also increase your bone density, pushing back against the harmful effects of conditions like osteoporosis and reducing the risk of a fracture or broken bone.

Other benefits of these exercises may not be so readily apparent, but it is easy to notice these improvements when you are looking for them. Strength training improves your coordination so you can manage complex physical tasks with little issue. You get used to performing the exercises by treating your body as a cohesive unit, and your balance improves. This also results in better posture, which alleviates tension in zones like your lower back and shoulders. Frequent strength training can also leave you feeling more energetic than usual. You may be able to accomplish more each day simply because you took a half hour or so to exercise, which is certainly a worthwhile investment.

Resistance training can also directly improve your physical health, lessening the effects of various health conditions. In some cases, regular workouts that involve strength exercises can reduce blood pressure and blood sugar levels, as your body metabolizes the excess glucose and regular exercise keeps your arteries clear of blockages. They may also improve your ability to manage chronic conditions like arthritis and diabetes, especially when it comes to pain relief. Additionally, while strength exercises may not explicitly target cardiovascular health, they can still contribute to heart health, and can lower your risk of a heart attack or stroke. In short, regular exercise is key, and strength training exercises are a great way to keep yourself in good shape.

One of the most important benefits of strength training for people with limited mobility is reducing the likelihood of injury from otherwise minor accidents. Stronger muscles are better able to support your joints. This means fewer falls, and if you do fall, there is less of a risk of experiencing a severe injury, as your muscles will help protect and cushion your bones.

These extensive benefits are only possible if you work out on a regular basis, which is why it is so important for seniors and others with limited mobility to remain active. Make sure to perform strength exercises that address the needs of your upper body and lower body as well as your core, though it is a good idea to take breaks in between focusing on each area of your body. With lots of exercise and plenty of time for resting and recovery, you are sure to find that the advantages of working out far outweigh any minor inconveniences that might have previously held you back.

Upper Body

While it is good practice to always lift from the legs when you are picking up especially heavy objects, this does not mean you should let your arms and shoulders fall by the wayside. If your lower back muscles must pick up the slack, you run a far greater risk of injury from putting too much of a strain on this sensitive area. Regular upper body exercise can alleviate this strain, eliminating pain and avoiding any injuries that would have otherwise been caused by overuse.

Upper body strength workouts incorporate a wide variety of exercises that target different muscle regions. Make sure to work your trapezius, deltoids, pectorals, triceps, biceps, and more when you are creating your daily, weekly, and monthly workout plans.

Wrist Curls

You have many delicate bones in your wrists, and if you do not have the appropriate amount of muscle, something as small as accidentally banging your arm against the table could cause a fracture. These wrist curls help develop these muscles so you can keep yourself safe while also getting stronger.

1. Grab a pair of water weights. Start with light weights and work your way up to heavier ones once you have tried the exercise out a few times.

2. Stand far enough away from the edge of the pool that you can freely move your arms without bumping the wall. If you need some support, you can turn away from the edge and lean back against it as long as you can still bring your arms down to your sides.

3. Hold the weights in your hands with your palms facing down. Straighten your arms and hold them out in front of you.

4. Without moving the rest of your body, roll your wrists down to push the weights just under the water's surface. Hold this position for a moment, feeling the tension, then roll your wrists back to the starting position and repeat.

Arm Rotations

Arm rotations primarily target your shoulder muscles. While holding your arms out to the side may not be too difficult at first, keeping them suspended and moving your arms in circles is a surprisingly effective exercise. Better yet, you can do these anywhere, whether you are in the pool or on dry land.

1. Stand in water that is about shoulder deep.

2. Stretch your arms out to either side of you. They should rest at or near the surface of the water .

3. Start rotating your arms, first making tiny circles. Then expand the diameter of your circles into medium-sized circles and then, finally, large circles. If you find that this is a little too strenuous, you can stick to small and medium circles at a slower pace.

4. As you perform these arm rotations, the top part of the circle should be above the water, while the bottom part should be underneath it. This means you do not want to go too fast, as you will likely exhaust your arms too quickly and splash yourself. Instead, maintain a steady pace and try to minimize the resulting splash.

5. Circle your arms forward several times and then backward several times as you progress through each size circle. After about 20 seconds going in one direction, switch to going the other way. This will help prevent soreness and improve your stamina.

Various Curls

A curl is a type of exercise that involves repetitive arm movements. They typically require the use of a weight, such as a dumbbell, to add resistance. Curls make for excellent tools in your workout toolbelt because they are extremely versatile. You can target different areas of your arms with different styles, such as your biceps, triceps, and shoulders. The targeted area depends on various factors including the direction of your palms while holding the weights and how you move your arms during the exercise.

Here, we will cover three different kinds of curls you can perform in the pool with water dumbbells. These curls help build strength in the fronts of your upper arms, your lower arms, and the backs of your upper arms, including the shoulder areas. You can include each of these options in your regular workout routines, but it might be a good idea to take at least a one-day break from arm workouts in between trying different kinds of curls, so you do not overwork your muscles.

Curls for the Front Muscles of the Upper Arms

The largest muscle in the front of your upper arm is your bicep. This is the muscle you can see under the skin if you flex your arm. Larger biceps indicate a more muscular physique and greater strength, so if you find your biceps to be a little lacking, try these curls.

1. Start your exercise by moving to an area of the pool where the water comes up to about elbow height.

2. Hold a weight in each of your hands. Wrap your fingers around the bar in the center of each water dumbbell.

3. Tuck your arms close to your sides, bending them at the elbow. Your lower arms should rest on the surface of the water. If the water level is a little higher or lower, then your elbows can be just above or below the surface respectively so long as you are holding your lower arms parallel to the ground.

4. Turn your arms so your palms are facing down toward the pool.

5. Press your lower arms down, bringing the weights underwater until they reach your thighs. Try to keep your elbows up against your torso and avoid bowing them outward as you push the weights down.

6. Next, bring the weights back up to the surface, but watch your form. You do not want to release all the tension at once and let the weights float back up on their own. Instead, maintain control and slowly bring your arms back up. Ensure your palms are facing down throughout the entire exercise.

7. Repeat for a full set of reps.

Curls for the Lower Arms

If you want to target your lower arms rather than your upper arms, all you need to do is hold the weights differently. By turning your palms upward instead of down toward the surface of the water, you shift the tension to the muscles in your forearms. While these muscles may not be as large as biceps or triceps, there are a lot of moving parts in your forearms, so it is important to build up your muscles to protect yourself from injury.

1. Stand in water that comes up to your elbows. Put your feet together for this exercise.

2. Hold a weight in each hand.

3. Bring your elbows in so they are close to your sides. Bend them at a 90-degree angle so your forearms are flat and parallel with the surface of the water.

4. Turn your wrists so you are holding the weights with your palms facing up toward the sky.

5. With your elbows bent and still tucked in against your sides, move your forearms to submerge the weights underwater. Pull them down so they are flush with your thighs.

6. Keep a solid grip on the weights allowing the natural water tension to control the force of movement. Slowly raise them back up to the surface, controlling their progression and keeping your palms in the same upward-facing position.

7. Repeat the lower arm curls to complete the set.

Curls for the Shoulders and Backs of the Arms

Muscles in your arms that are involved in lifting up heavy objects include your trapezius or traps in your shoulder and your triceps in the backs of your arms. Every part of your

101

upper body works together as you exercise and move through daily life, so be sure to pay these muscle groups some attention with curls as well.

1. Sit down on the steps of the pool, submerging yourself deep enough that the water rises to your chest. Turn your body a little to the side.

2. Straighten your back and bring your legs together in front of you in a relaxed seated position.

3. If you are turned toward the left, hold a weight in your right hand. If you are turned toward the right, hold the weight with your left hand. Make sure you can move your arm and the weight far enough back behind and in front of you without bumping into anything, such as the step, a railing, or the wall of the pool. If not, turn further until you can move freely.

4. Bring the arm holding the weight in toward your side, bending it at the elbow. Keep the arm at this 90-degree angle throughout the entire exercise. Maintaining good form is especially important when targeting specific muscle groups.

5. You want your palm to face down toward your leg.

6. Rotate your shoulder to move your elbow behind you. Only move as far as is comfortable for you.

7. While keeping control of the weight, bring your arm back to the starting position. Double check that your palm is still facing toward your leg.

8. Repeat this movement, completing multiple reps.

9. When you have finished a full set with one arm, turn to the opposite side, switch arms, and repeat the workout once again on the other side of your body.

Inverted Arm Lifts to the Sides

When you are exercising above ground, you typically raise dumbbells up into the air, as you work against gravity. In the water, this movement gets inverted. Instead, you will need to push the weights down, working against the resistance of the water and the flotation devices. These inverted arm lifts make great use of this reversion to give you an excellent work out of your arms, shoulders, back, and neck muscles.

1. Stand in the deep end of the pool. Go far enough that the water comes up to and submerges your shoulders, but make sure you can keep your chin above water without issue.

2. Hold a weight in each hand and raise your arms out to your sides as if resting on the surface of the water.

3. Turn your palms so they face down toward the bottom of the pool. As you perform the exercise, they will point toward your body.

4. Keeping your arms straight, swing them down and bring them in toward your thighs. You should be able to touch your thighs with the weights, but if not, just go as far as you can.

5. Hold this for a moment, then return your arms to the starting position. Maintain control of your movement the whole time, and do not allow the weights to float back up to the surface on their own.

6. Repeat the exercise.

Inverted Arm Lifts to the Front

In this exercise, you will follow the steps to the inverted arm lifts to the sides, but you will be bringing the weights in front of you instead. This addition works the rotator cuffs in your arms as well as chest muscles like your pectorals, or pecs for short. Like the previous exercise, you will be working against the buoyancy of the weights, which provides the perfect level of tension for muscle growth without strain.

1. Stand up straight in the water. Move to a deep enough area of the pool that your shoulders are submerged but your chin is comfortably above the water's surface.

2. Stretch your arms out in front of you, keeping them on the surface of the water.

3. Hold a weight in each hand. Rotate your arms so your palms face down toward the bottom of the pool.

4. Take a deep breath in and push the weights down below the surface. Try to bring them all the way down until they brush your thighs, keeping your arms straight as you go.

5. Hold, then release the breath and steadily bring the weights back up to the surface. Again, you want to maintain tight control over them so you can keep your arms straight and avoid jerky movements.

6. Repeat the exercise as many times as desired.

Inverted Push-Ups

As you might imagine, it is a little difficult to perform regular push-ups when you are in the water. Since gravity is not weighing you down the same way, you might struggle to lower yourself to the floor of the pool, and you would have to submerge your head to maintain proper form. Inverted push-ups allow you gain similar results while working within the boundaries of a pool environment. By using the pool stairs, you can dip yourself down with your arms, achieving a similar kind of exercise that is especially effective for strengthening your triceps.

1. Sit down on one of the pool steps. Your feet should rest comfortably and flat on the bottom of the pool, and the water should come up to about your midsection.

2. Rest the palms of your hands on the step next to you, bracketing your legs. Keep your hands facing forward. You can curl your fingers around the edge of the step.

3. Push down with your hands to raise your torso into the water. You may need to lean back a little as you lift so you can fully raise your torso up off the step. Make sure you are stable enough to support yourself before you proceed.

4. Keep your palms on the step, then swing your buttocks out toward your feet. It should be just past the edge of the pool step so you can dip down without bumping against anything.

5. Bend your arms to lower the weight of your torso down a few inches. Then straighten your arms to lift

yourself back up. It helps to breathe in as you dip down and breathe back out as you rise up.

6. Repeat the inverted push-up to finish the set.

Lower Body

Your lower body is the main area involved in movement and support. Strengthening your lower body allows you to improve your balance steadily over time, which means you will feel more stable as you move around throughout your day. The more you exercise the various muscle groups in your lower body, the less likely it is that you will fall and hurt yourself, which means you can look and feel more confident every day. Significant muscle groups in your lower body include your glutes in your buttocks, your quadriceps, or quads in the front of your thighs, your hamstrings in the back of your thighs, and your calves.

Lift on Toes

You may have trouble lifting yourself up on your toes when you are trying to grab something off a high shelf at home but performing this exercise in the pool is much easier. As you build up your calves and the muscles near your ankles, you will find that this motion becomes far less difficult. This exercise has the added benefit of reducing the risk of ankle fractures and sprains as well.

1. Stand in waist-deep water. Hold your arms out in front of you and place your feet shoulder-width apart. If you find you need a little more support as you perform this

exercise, you can try loosely holding onto the edge of the pool or a flotation device.

2. Shift your weight forward lifting your weight up onto the balls of your feet, then onto your toes, (if you are able). Only lift yourself up by a few inches. If you cannot fully raise your arches off the bottom of the pool yet, at least try to lift your heels.

3. Hold this position for a few seconds.

4. Slowly lower yourself back toward the ground. Remember to shift your weight back to center as you move.

5. If you want to add a little challenge to this workout, bring your feet together and then raise and lower yourself. This provides more of a challenge for balancing and engages your core in addition to your lower body.

6. Repeat the exercise as desired.

Leg Lift

Leg lifts allow you to target many different muscles in your lower body. The standard leg lift works the joints in your hips and engages your quads and glutes. It also supports the further development of your balance, as you will be lifting one leg at a time. With additions, you can also target the muscles near your shins and in your calves. Leg lifts are a very simple exercise, but the many variations you can perform means they will always have a spot in your workout routine.

1. Face the edge of the pool and hold onto it. Stand up straight and tall, relaxing your shoulders.

2. While keeping your legs straight, shift your weight to your left leg and lift your right leg out to the side and up towards the surface of the water. You should be lifting your foot at least a few inches off the ground. If you are struggling, put a little more weight on the edge of the pool to help you lift yourself up but only lift as high as you are comfortable.

3. Hold this a moment, then return your foot to the floor of the pool.

4. Complete a full set with one leg, then swap to the other leg and repeat the exercise. (A set consists of however many repetitions you are comfortable doing.)

5. To make the workout even more effective, point your feet and toes as you raise each leg. This works the muscles along your shins.

6. If you rotate your foot so it is flat, you can work your calf muscles as well.

7. You can work both sets of muscles in the shins and calves if you alternate your foot from pointed to flexed as you lift and lower your leg.

8. Try lifting each leg a bit higher to add a little more challenge.

9. You can also increase the intensity by tying a pool noodle into a knot, slipping it around your ankle, and then doing the leg lifts. This adds resistance and

tension. You can achieve a similar effect with an aquatic ankle weight.

Buttocks Crunch

Your glutes are essential muscles for movement and support. They assist in supporting the weight of your upper body and developing your glute strength comes with a number of other positive effects. They can alleviate pain from your hips and lower back, and they are a great way to improve your posture and balance as a result. These buttocks crunches help you build your muscles in your glutes as well as your hamstrings, all without engaging in more exhausting and difficult exercises like split squats and regular crunches.

1. Hold onto the edge of the pool for support.

2. Rest your feet flat on the bottom of the pool and bring them together. Stand up straight, dropping your shoulders and maintaining good posture with your back.

3. While keeping your legs straightened, move one leg back a few inches off the ground behind you. You should be able to feel the tension in the muscles in your buttocks. If not, raise your leg a little higher behind you as you flex your glutes.

4. Hold this pose for a moment, then lower your leg back to the ground.

5. Complete a full set of reps with one leg, then switch to your other leg.

6. There are a few ways to increase the level of challenge of this exercise. Start by just lifting your leg higher and higher with each rep. You should never feel any discomfort but raising your leg further will deepen your stretch and better target your leg and glute muscles.

7. Add more resistance by tying a pool noodle into a knot and slipping it around your ankle. When you raise your leg, you will need to work harder to push back against the added water tension. You can also use ankle weights that are specially designed for use in the water.

Crouching With Weights

Kneeling down in the water can be a fairly decent workout on its own. As you sink down, you are pushing against water tension while also engaging the muscles in the front and back of your legs. You get a similarly effective workout from rising back up out of the kneeling position. When you add weights to the mix, you make this exercise even more effective. You will need to push the weights down while also moving your body down into the water yourself, meaning you are targeting multiple zones of your body. Kneeling with weights is best performed in the shallow end of the pool, so you do not have to be a very experienced swimmer to enjoy the benefits of this exercise.

1. Hold a weight in each hand. Turn your arms so your palms face inward toward your body.

2. Stand with your feet together and your arms held loosely at your sides. You should stand in water that is

shallow enough that you do not have to exert much force to keep the weights in this position. Ideally, they should be resting just below the surface of the water. Additionally, keep your back as straight as possible.

3. Without moving the rest of your body, bend your knees so you can sink down into the water keeping your back as straight as possible. Kneel down as far as you are comfortable going. Make sure you can complete the exercise without submerging your face.

4. As you kneel, hold your arms straight at your sides, pushing the weights down. You should be able to feel the added tension up your arms as you move.

5. Hold for a moment at the lowest point, then slowly raise yourself back up, keeping tight control of the weights so they do not jerk your arms up too fast.

6. Repeat the exercise until you reach your desired repetitions to complete the set.

Lunge With Weights

This exercise is similar to the previous one, but you will only have to bend one leg at a time. This may be a little easier for you if you experience joint stiffness in your legs which would otherwise prevent you from fully kneeling down in the water. Performing lunges in the pool is often easier than performing them above ground, as the water takes some of the pressure off your joints. As a result, these lunges are a great way to engage your lower body without tiring yourself out or straining yourself.

1. Begin by moving to the shallow end of the pool, where this exercise is best performed.

2. Hold a weight in each hand and let your arms fall to rest at your sides.

3. Turn your hands so your palms face your legs. Then take a step forward with one leg so you are in a staggered stance. Keep your back as straight as possible in this starting pose and throughout the exercise. This will help you get an especially deep stretch when you lunge.

4. Bend both knees to lunge down as far as is comfortable for you. Your legs should ideally be bent at 90-degree angles, with the thigh of your front leg parallel to the ground, but you may not be able to dip down this far just yet.

5. As you lower yourself down into the lunge, keep your arms straight down at your sides. You will need to push down to hold them in place as you submerge the weights.

6. Slowly stand back up again, keeping your movements relaxed and gradual.

7. Repeat the exercise, keeping your legs in the same position to finish the set.

8. Take a brief break, then switch the position of your feet. Repeat the exercise to work the opposite side of your body.

Bicycle or Twist in the Corner of the Pool

This exercise is a little more difficult than some of the other ones we have covered so far, but it provides a great challenge if you are up to it. You will need to be able to support most of your weight on your arms, so it is best to only perform this exercise on days where your arms are not feeling sore or stiff. Even though this is primarily a lower body workout, it also targets your triceps and traps, making for an incredibly effective overall workout.

There are two ways to perform this exercise. The first involves moving your legs like you are pedaling a bicycle, while the second involves twisting your hips and legs from side to side. You can just choose one of these depending on what you feel up to on any given day, or you can attempt to perform both in succession for a truly deep lower body workout.

1. Move to the corner of the pool and turn so your back is facing the intersection of the walls. This exercise is best performed in the deep end, as you will want to keep your body mostly submerged (with the water covering your shoulders but not your chin or head) and the shallow end may not allow for this. Make sure you are comfortable swimming before attempting to move into the deepest part of the pool.

2. Stretch your arms out to your sides and rest them on the edges of the pool behind you. You will need to hold on while performing the exercise, which means you will need to find a comfortable position that allows you to support your body weight or lift your upper body out of the water without too much strain. You can try

a few different poses until you find one that works, as the best pose will vary depending on your height and weight. You may need to lean back further, turn your hands forward or backward, or adjust the amount of bend in your arms.

3. Lift your legs off the floor of the pool, primarily by supporting your body weight with your arms. Lift your legs up in front of you so you are in a seated position while floating in the water. If needed, stand up to adjust your grip on the edge of the pool to stabilize yourself.

4. Exercise using either the bicycle or twist method, as outlined here:

    a. Bicycling:

        i. Pump your legs in a circular motion, alternating them like you are pushing down on the pedals of a bicycle. You can twist your torso a little as you move for a deeper stretch but try to keep your arms and neck as still as possible to prevent unnecessary strain.

    b. Twist:

        i. Keep your legs together and bent in the seated position. Then twist from the hips, turning to the right. Hold this pose, return to the center, and twist to the left. Continue repeating these twists, making sure your knees remain together throughout, and taking breaks as needed.

5. Note that it can be difficult to keep yourself supported while doing either of these exercises. It is okay to

perform fewer reps than usual and to let yourself rest for a while in between sets. You will steadily improve your endurance over time.

6. Whatever motion you choose can be performed as quickly or as slowly as your body permits. Try starting slow and working your way up to faster movements, or alternatively, really slow down and feel the contraction of each muscle as you move.

Core Body

A great deal of your strength comes not from your arms or your legs but from your core. Strong core muscles help you stave off fatigue as you perform other exercises, especially cardiovascular exercises. They can also help reduce your risk of injury and improve your overall health while supporting the rest of your body.

View your core not just as its own group of muscles, but also as the connection between the upper and lower halves of your body. Most exercises involve engaging your core in some way, even if it is just tensing your abs to keep yourself stable during your workout. Therefore, you want to keep this area as strong as possible so you can continue to strengthen the rest of your body.

Typical above ground core exercises include high-intensity and often fairly difficult exercises like crunches, bridges, and extended planks. You may have trouble holding these poses or completing multiple reps if you have weakened or swollen joints. Performing alternate core exercises in the water, like inverted sit-ups and arm butterflies, are much more accessible to people with limited mobility. These workouts offer a great way to strengthen your core without the risk of overtaxing yourself, so be sure to frequently incorporate them into your regular routine.

Arm Swing

The arm swing exercise targets your abs and obliques, which are the muscles that run along the sides of your abdomen. Twisting to the left works your right obliques, while twisting to the right works the left obliques. This is why it is so important to ensure you are getting a nice even workout on each side with an equal number of reps, as you do not want to end up lopsided.

This exercise can be performed in either waist-deep or chest-deep water. In waist-deep water, your arms are above the surface, which makes the exercise a little easier but may aggravate your joints a bit more. Exercising in chest-deep water means your arms are mostly submerged, which makes the exercise more difficult but also lessens the risk of jarring your joints, as the water reduces the impact. Choose the depth that works best for your body and your needs.

1. Find a depth you are comfortable with in the pool. Extend both of your arms out in front of you with your palms facing each other.

2. You can either keep your palms about the same distance apart throughout the exercise or clasp them together if you want to ensure your arms do not move too far apart. Then swing your arms over to the right, going as far as you can before returning them to the center.

116

3. Repeat the process, this time swinging your arms to the left. Continue until you have completed a full set.

Inverted Sit-Up

The inverted sit up is similar to the inverted push-up, as it takes a more difficult exercise and makes it easier by using the pool to your advantage. In the inverted sit-up, you sit on the steps and bend down instead of curling your body up, pushing the weights underwater to add tension. This is much more accessible than trying to lift up your whole-body weight, and it offers many of the same health benefits as you're working to strengthen your muscles.

1. Sit down on the middle step of the pool. You should be able to rest your feet comfortably on the floor white still having most of your chest out of the water. Sit with your legs together in front of you.

2. Hold a weight in each hand. Turn your palms so they are facing toward your thighs.

3. Straighten your arms. Move the weights so they bracket your knees. They should hang off the edge of the seat of the pool.

4. Bend at the waist and lean toward the water while still keeping yourself stable. Hold your arms straight as you bend down, pushing on the weights so they continue to sink down before the surface of the water. Make sure to keep your head above the water during this exercise.

5. Maintain control over the momentum of the weights as you lean backward and return to the starting position.

117

6. Repeat the exercise. Make sure to limit the movement of your arms, as this is not an upper body workout. This will allow you to get a deeper workout in your abs and back muscles, strengthening your core.

Arm Butterflies

The arm butterfly exercise is named after the motion your arms make while performing it. You will need to stretch them out to your sides and back, almost like the flapping of butterfly wings. While this exercise does involve some muscles in your upper body, it is primarily a workout for your chest and lower back muscles, as these big, slow-paced arm movements compress and stress the muscles in your torso and core area. Maintaining good form is especially important when performing arm butterflies, so periodically double check that you are following the motions right and make adjustments if necessary.

1. Go deep enough into the pool that the water fully covers your shoulders, but make sure to keep your chin above the surface. You want to be able to breathe easily. If you are not comfortable in the deep end just yet, you can also achieve this by sitting on the bottom step of the pool, as long as your head is still above the water.

2. Hold a weight in each hand. It is a good idea to use heavier weights for this exercise, as the movements are slow, and the added weight will ensure you are really engaging your core when you move your arms.

3. Bend your elbows slightly, then reach your arms out in front of you with your palms facing toward each other.

118

Your forearms should be positioned in front of your chest.

4. Without fully straightening your arms, move them out to your sides until they are almost in line with either side of your body. If you feel comfortable doing so, you can even extend your arms a little behind your back by rotating at the elbows.

5. Ensure your arms remain just below the surface of the water as you repeat these movements, bringing your arms back in front of you and out to the sides again at a slow, measured pace.

6. With each set, you should feel the muscles in your chest and back getting a workout. If not, try exaggerating your motions, bringing your arms tighter together in front of you and spreading them out further on either side of you.

Noodle Lean or Twists

Pool noodles are most commonly used for recreation when swimming, but they can be very versatile when you are exercising in the pool too. You can perform noodle leans and twists with them, both of which engage your core muscles including your abs and your obliques. This is a great inexpensive way to work out if you are not ready to commit to buying a whole set of water weights and other kinds of equipment, as pool noodles are cheap and easy to use.

1. Hold your arms out in front of you and grab the ends of the pool noodle in your hands. Curve the noodle up

so it is bent in an arc or rainbow-like shape, and make sure you have a firm grip on the ends of the noodle.

2. Raise the pool noodle above the water and into the air over your head. From here, you can perform two different exercises depending on the intensity and the type of workout you are looking for.

   a. While keeping the pool noodle above your head, lean your body to the left, going as far as you can without falling into the water. Then return to the center and lean to the right. These noodle leans work the muscles along the sides of your ribs, stretching and compressing them for a serious workout without any risk of impact-related injury.

   b. Rather than leaning from side to side, twist your torso in each direction. Again, move slowly and really feel the pull and push of your muscles. This works not only your obliques, but also your abs and back muscles, which makes it a great way to relieve back tension.

No matter what kind of stretch exercises you perform, know that you are supporting your physical wellbeing as you complete them. Just a few strength exercises incorporated into your workout routine can work wonders for your fitness, level of mobility, and ability to manage chronic pain. These exercises may not seem especially strenuous compared to the heavy weightlifting some gym-goers do, but you do not have to hold yourself to such a high standard. Perform the exercises you are capable of doing and you will find that these low-impact workouts will make all the difference in keeping you healthy and happy.

CHAPTER 11

Sample Workouts

In chapters five and six, we looked at some of the basic parts of a well-rounded workout, as well as good practices for creating and sticking to your own exercise routine. Now that you know the kinds of exercises you can perform in the pool, you can start to decide which exercises you are interested in, which ones you are capable of performing with good form, and how you are going to maintain your commitment to working out on a regular basis.

Creating the perfect workout plan for your abilities and needs is important when you are trying to keep yourself motivated to exercise routinely. Your plan should be tailored to suit your individual body. You will not do yourself any favors if you try to push yourself too hard, purposefully ignoring your limitations and likely ending up demotivated or even injured as a result. At the same time, you want to avoid creating a workout routine that is too sparse, as you will hardly feel any benefits this way. Another pitfall to avoid is loading up on too many exercises that target the same muscle groups. While toning your abs is good, this should not come at the expense of strengthening your arms and legs or doing some cardio occasionally. The best workouts cycle through different areas of your body, ensuring you spend enough time on each one so you can look and feel your best.

At first, it may be a little difficult to plan your own workout, especially if you have never really gotten serious about exercise before. You might not know how intense is too intense, or you could be unsure about which exercises pair together well. While you will come to understand all of this with time and practice, it is okay to be unsure right now, as you are just starting out. In this chapter, we will look at some sample workouts you can try out and see if they work for you. Pay attention to how you feel afterward, especially in regard to soreness and stiffness. You can adjust these sample workouts as needed once you get a good idea of what kind of exercises you should be performing and where your personal limits are. Use them as a blueprint to create a unique, personalized routine just for you.

Sample Upper Body Workouts

Warm-Up and Cooldown

When creating a warm-up plan, consider what exercises you are going to perform, and make sure to target these areas. You can also add some unstructured stretches if you feel like any areas are still tense. Stretch the muscles in your arms, upper back, neck, and the rest of your upper body with these warm-up and cooldown exercises:

- Finger walks
- Wrist rolls

- Upper arm stretches

Exercises

You have now warmed yourself up and are ready to start moving your arms. Select some low-impact pool exercises to work with from those listed in chapters eight and ten, or use the following workout plan:

- Wrist curls

- Curls for the lower arms

- Curls for the shoulders and backs of the arms

Remember to perform the same exercises you used to warm up as your cooldown once you are done exercising. Take breaks as needed, and pace yourself appropriately.

Here is another set of warm-ups, cooldowns, and exercises you can use if you decide the first workout is not for you, or if you want to switch things up.

Warm-Up and Cooldown

- Lower arm stretches

- Lean and stand

- Shoulder and arm stretch

Exercises

- Inverted push-ups

- Inverted arm lifts to the front

The list of exercises is a little shorter in this workout because the selected exercises are somewhat more intense. You do not want to exhaust yourself, so it is best to do only a few of the more strenuous exercises, or to pair one strenuous workout with one or two less intense ones.

Sample Lower Body Workout

Lower body warm-ups, cooldowns, and exercises target many different muscles in your lower waist area, your legs, and your feet. Make sure you get in a good stretch first, as these muscles are prone to cramping, and they can remain sore for days or even weeks after a workout if you do not prepare yourself properly. Try to include some activity for all muscle groups in your lower body, including your glutes, hamstrings, quads, calves, feet, and hips.

Here are two workout options that address the fitness needs of your lower body. You can choose the one that suits you best, or swap between one workout and the other depending on what you feel like doing each day.

Warm-Up and Cooldown

- Toe points
- Lunges to stretch calves
- Knee lifts

Exercises

- Leg lifts

- Lunge with weights
- Lift on toes

This set of exercises and stretches is a little less intense. If you are looking for a challenge, try the second workout plan.

Warm-Up and Cooldown

- Toe points
- Hip swings
- Front of the thigh stretch

Exercises

- Kneel with weights
- Buttocks crunches
- Bicycle or twist in the corner of the pool

Sample Core Body or Cardio Workout

Due to how taxing core and cardio focused workouts can be on your system, you may want to limit yourself on how many you perform on a given day. Many cardio workouts engage your core muscles and vice versa, so you can rest assured you are not missing out on anything by combining these two types of workouts. Warming up and cooling down is especially important for both core and cardio exercises, so take care to perform enough sets and reps that you feel sufficiently limber before you start on the exercises.

Warm-Up and Cooldown

- Toe point
- Lunge
- Hip swing

Exercises

- Walking

This is a low-intensity workout that does not put too much strain on your body. It is perfect for when you are just starting out. As you get acclimated, you start feeling ready for a more challenging workout, try out the second selection of warm-ups and exercises.

Warm-Up and Cooldown

- Lean and stand
- Knee lifts
- Front of the thigh stretches
- Boxer punches if you swing your arms while jogging

For this set of exercises, you will also want to add on some arm stretches. These can be as simple as reaching your arms out to the sides or up above your head, or something more complex like the upper and lower arm stretches.

Exercises

- Bunny hops

- Jogging

In addition to a regular jog, you can also incorporate boxer punches into this exercise for an added workout. Instead of letting your arms swing, bring them up like you are guarding your torso, and shadow box as you jog through the water. This increases your heart rate and engages your core. It can also help loosen some of the muscles that would normally become tight when you are going for a jog.

Sample Overall Body Workout

Some days, you may want to target specific areas of your body. Other days, you may find it more beneficial to perform a full body workout that addresses many areas at the same time. There are many ways to mix and match workouts that engage muscles from all over your body, so feel free to experiment and come up with a workout plan that works for you. Since you can use just about any exercises, try mixing things up every time you have an overall body workout day as a nice change of pace. Just make sure that your warm-up and cooldown cover all your different muscle groups as well and stretch yourself out sufficiently before you get started.

I think the next 4 sections should have a heading differentiation. Maybe Set 1 and Set 2?(I would probably go with 1 overall heading like Possible set options for workouts)

Warm-Up and Cooldown

- Boxer punches

- Knee lifts

- Core rotations

Exercises

- Inverted push-ups

- Bicycle or twist in the corner of the pool

- Arm butterflies

Warm-Up and Cooldown

- Shoulder and upper arm stretches

- Hip swings

- Chest stretches

Exercises

- Inverted arm lifts to the front

- Kneel with weights

- Inverted sit-ups

Be sure to take things nice and slow with plenty of breaks when you are performing an overall body workout. You do not want to exhaust yourself, and it's easy to get carried away with planning to tackle far more exercises than you could reasonably complete. This is an easy way to leave yourself sore and unwilling to continue working out. If you pace yourself and pay attention to what your body is telling you, you can complete a great overall body workout without any issues.

Again, feel free to adjust anything in this set of workouts to suit your needs, just as you can change any of the workout plans listed in this chapter. They are merely suggestions to get you started on the right path. As you turn exercise into a regular occurrence and you steadily build up your muscles over time, you will get a better sense of what your body is capable of and what kinds of exercises you are interested in performing, which will result in a more effective and fulfilling personalized workout.

Conclusion

The greatest obstacle to change is often your own tendency to resist it. It is very easy to continue living as you have been for years, regardless of the negative consequences. If you struggle with mobility, whether it is the result of your age, a health condition, or an injury, it is tempting to give up on exercise entirely. There is very little stopping you from deciding that it is too difficult for you, and you are not going to give any of the exercises in this book a try. However, if you do this, you are denying yourself the chance to drastically improve your physical health, manage chronic pain, alleviate soreness, and improve your overall wellbeing.

Exercise is important for everyone regardless of how old, young, fit, or out of shape you are. Just by getting your body moving, even a little bit with gentle, low-impact exercises, you can enjoy several benefits that will improve your quality of life. You will strengthen your muscles and improve your cardiovascular health over time, which can help you improve your mobility, posture, and balance. This reduces the risk of suffering a major injury from a fall or minor accident. On top of this, when you look for creative ways to get moving, such as exercising in the pool, you can make exercise fun. With so many reasons to start working out, there is no excuse to not try. The only one who can stand in your way is yourself.

As you work up the nerve to start exercising, or if you ever start to doubt yourself and want to give up, remind yourself that you can do this! It does not matter if you are a professional athlete or someone who has rarely, if ever, exercised before now. As long as you have access to a pool and you can swim, you can try out these exercises. Each exercise is designed to be easy for anyone to complete, and you can make adjustments as needed if you struggle with any of them. These are doable movements, and the results are more than worth the time and energy you will invest into yourself when you get in the pool.

Give yourself the chance you need to succeed. Believe in your own physical abilities. Try to stick to a workout routine a few times a week and give yourself a month or two to get used to it before you give yourself a chance to quit. Then, once you have given it a fair shot, consider how much progress you have made and how you feel. Ask yourself questions like, "Does this feel like work?", "Do I enjoy it?", "Am I able to move better?", and "Do I feel better?" Your answers just might surprise you, but you will not know for sure unless you give it a shot.

With low-impact swimming pool exercises, you can not only look better, but also feel better. Working out for even two or three days a week will allow you to always be at your best, and that is exactly what you deserve. When you invest in yourself through exercise, you give yourself the opportunity to improve. You are worth the effort, so do not delay. Get in the pool today, and with some time and effort, you will be amazed at the incredible results.

Our Thing Media, LLC

If you would like to hear about other books we are publishing, feel free to sign up for our newsletter by submitting your email address here: https://ourthingmedia.activehosted.com/f/1. You can unsubscribe at any time. (Please know that we will only use your email address to send a newsletter, it will never be sold or shared with anyone else.)

Do you want free books? If you become a member of the Our Thing Media review team, we will give you free books! We are always looking for honest opinions and feedback. This just means you get books for free and, in return, you give your feedback. That's it! (You can unsubscribe from this at any time.) To become part of our review team, submit your email address here: https://ourthingmedia.activehosted.com/f/3

Made in the USA
Monee, IL
08 July 2022